Positive Parenting

————— ❧☙❧☙ —————

Discover The Secrets To Raising
Happy, Healthy, And Loving
Children Without Breaking Their
Spirit

Natasha Becker

Copyright 2019 © Natasha Becker

Legal & Disclaimer

including specific information will be considered an illegal act irrespective of if it is done electronically or in print. This extends to creating a secondary or tertiary copy of the work or a recorded copy and is only allowed with an express written consent from the Publisher. All additional right reserved.

The information in the following pages is broadly considered to be a truthful and accurate account of facts, and as such any inattention, use or misuse of the information in question by the reader will render any resulting actions solely under their purview. There are no scenarios in which the publisher or the original author of this work can be in any fashion deemed liable for any hardship or damages that may befall them after undertaking information described herein.

Additionally, the information in the following pages is intended only for informational purposes and should thus be thought of as universal. As befitting its nature, it is presented without assurance regarding its prolonged validity or interim quality. Trademarks that are mentioned are done without written consent and can in no way be considered an endorsement from the trademark holder.

Table of Contents

Introduction

The act of parenting is a fundamental part of the human experience and the natural world as a whole. We see it right across the vast spectrum of the fauna that we share our planet with, from dedicated penguin fathers that carry and care for their unhatched young on top of their feet day and night to the single-minded devotion of octopus mothers that starve themselves to death to protect their spawn. There are few instincts more powerful than those that direct us to treat our young with committed and unconditional nurturing love. We feel an intense need to protect our vulnerable and innocent children and possess a great desire to raise and guide them as best we can.

If our intentions correlated perfectly with our actions, there wouldn't be a need for this book. Almost all of us want nothing but the best for our children, and if raising them well was as easy as simply wanting to, we'd live in a much better world. Unfortunately, things are far more complicated than that. When we try our best to teach our kids how to behave, how to be responsible and polite, we often find our words falling on deaf ears and the same lessons going unlearnt despite us trying our best to teach them, time after time. The difficulty in raising children is something that is often attributed to a 'kids these days' mentality, especially by older generations, who have forgotten what it was really like to be young and so wave their hands and say that today's children are out of control, selfish, lacking in respect, and that things were far better when they were young. This attitude is a tale as old as time. Raising children has always been, and will always be, a process that is far from easy. Kids can be hard work. It's just the nature of the job.

Parenting is one of the most difficult things you will ever have to do. It is also one of the most rewarding, enlightening, and beautiful experiences it is possible for you to have. Raising children to become independent, compassionate, happy, and thriving young adults can be an incredibly hard task even when you know how to do it in a positive and loving manner. When you're trapped by the limits of your own understanding, it can be almost impossible. It's all too easy to become frustrated and impatient and find yourself resorting to acting out of anger and resentment from sheer desperation. It doesn't have to be that way. This book is a guide that will teach you to follow a positive, productive, and effective path through the murky, confusing world of parenting, in order to encourage and support you in your role as a caregiver, teacher, entertainer, and friend to your children.

Positive parenting is a process. It's about far more than just learning the theories and ideas that surround it. It's a participatory experience that encourages you to broaden your understanding of yourself, others, and your children, and the incredible role that you play in their development from helpless newborns to a happy, healthy, well-adjusted young people. Parenting is a highly intuitive experience — you have to learn to trust your gut and your instincts. That's what this guide aims to do; it will instill a particular attitude and outlook within you that allows you to be an intuitive parent to your children in a positive way and make good decisions when situations arise that you need to respond to. When it comes to doing this, understanding is essential. You have to possess the knowledge about why positive parenting works before you can properly implement it into your family. You have to first learn to understand yourself in order to really come to understand your children. In order to look out, you must first look inwards. You have to be able to pause before you act and reflect on your own actions. No-one is perfect; having the self-awareness and honesty to admit your mistakes to yourself and your children will go a very, very long way towards cultivating a rewarding and positive relationship with them, as well as showing them the value of humility.

Like anything in life, the process of parenting is a journey. It will always have its ups and downs. Positive parenting isn't about being perfect, it's about recognizing that no matter what happens, the important thing is being able to calm down and take the time to think things through, and ensure that the right lessons are learned by everyone in your family. It's a long journey, so a great deal of patience and commitment will be required on your part. Luckily for you, the very fact that you're either going to be a parent or you're a parent already means that you're already committed to the longest of journeys; if you're doing it anyway, then you should do it properly. Take the lessons of this guide to heart. There will always be good days and bad days, times when you feel blessed to have the chance to witness the miracle and beauty of raising children for yourself, and times when you just want to give up and run away. This duality of life is something we all experience from time to time. It's just part of being human. You might want to scream and tear your hair out in desperation because of the frustration you feel after trying your best to make your kids be quiet, or eat their dinner, or go to sleep. It doesn't make you a bad person, and it doesn't make you a bad parent.

Whether you're picking this book up because you're going to be a parent soon or you're already years deep into the process and are looking for ideas and assistance, this book will take you through A-Z of positive parenting and provide you with the tools and understanding you need to guide you on your journey. It contains the raw information and background theories you need to get to grips with positive parenting as well as examples and exercises to help you more thoroughly apply what you've learned to your everyday life. This book is intended to supply you with the insight, attitude, and encouragement you need to help you fully embrace the beauty and fulfillment of being a parent. All it requires is that you keep an open mind and a willingness to try out techniques you might not be used to — especially if you were raised in a more traditional, authoritarian manner.

Positive parenting isn't about being 'soft', or 'weak' on your children, or allowing them to rule the roost. It's about approaching their development from a place of deep compassion and understanding for the struggles and obstacles they face, something that is sorely needed more than ever in this world. It can be easy to dismiss some problems children face because of their apparently trivial nature, but when we do this we disregard the fact that issues that may seem silly to us may well be one of the most difficult and stressful situations a child has encountered in their young lives. Boundaries and rules are important, as is enforcing them with the knowledge that everyone, including children, is usually just doing the best they can with the information they have at hand at any one time.

We're ruled by emotions and hormones. They cloud our judgment, frustrate us, and cause us to react with anger and hurt those we love the most in this world. Despite this, we have the ability to look back in retrospect and learn lessons from our past mistakes and misgivings. That, along with kindness, compassion, and a mindset that seeks to understand, rather than push away things that seem alien to us, is the essence of positive parenting. It's not just about the way you treat your children, but the way you treat other adults and yourself. It's impossible to raise your children in a positive manner when you have little positive regard for others or yourself. If you're impatient, have a short temper and are quick to react with anger to the inconveniences you face in your life, how can you expect to treat your children any differently? They can frustrate us far more and more often than bad drivers or when the grocery store is out of whatever you need. That's why positive parenting can be so difficult for people — it requires a great deal of patience, resistance to inconvenience, and understanding of the self and others to be effectively practiced.

With this in mind, let's dive into the thick of the middle of parenting and begin the journey of learning how to do it in a more positive manner.

Part One:

The Positive Parenting Theory

The Positive Parenting Theory refers to a movement that has been gaining momentum in recent years regarding the way in which parents raise their children.

An Overview Of The Positive Parenting Theory

I t's becoming more and more common, and it's resulting in increasing numbers of well-raised, emotionally stable, kind, compassionate young adults. Positive parenting is an entire approach to parenting built on ideas which would have seemed radical just a few decades ago, but with time and progress have come to be widely accepted and practiced by people determined to raise their children as well as they can. It represents a total departure from more traditional, fear-based parenting techniques that emphasize children being raised to be unquestioningly obedient and compliant through a parental style characterized by strict discipline, punishment, and hard-taught lessons that 'will do them good in the long run'.

Positive parenting shrugs off this traditional style in favor of an approach that is centered on parents cultivating loving, cooperative relationships with their children, based upon a deep respect for their individuality and autonomy as people. Essentially, it involves recoiling against the notion that a child's wants and needs are irrelevant and secondary to those of adults. Instead, positive parenting embraces the potential for a parent to guide and develop their child in an accommodating, thoroughly involved, and interesting manner. Rather than revolving around power struggles, control, and the assertion of dominance, positive parenting entails fostering an attitude of equality between all the members of the family. Everyone matters exactly the same amount, everyone is allowed to speak their mind, and everyone is treated as a completely individual person, regardless of their age.

The theory of positive parenting is very different from how the majority of children have been raised throughout recorded history. It's a fundamental, radical overhaul in how children are treated and spoken to, how their behavior is corrected, and even how they are thought about by their parents. It consists of alternative ways of approaching the entire parent-child relationship in order to shape and mold children in a more positive and beneficial way, using very different tactics that seek to develop much stronger, more loving bonds between parents and children. For example, rather than reacting to misbehavior with an immediate negative response borne out of frustration — such as shouting — positive parenting instead substitutes in the practice of engaging a misbehaving child in a way that appeals to them; maintaining a patient, understanding tone of voice, and approaching the problem with a careful consideration of the circumstances of the situation. Perhaps the child is bored, or tired, or hungry, or overly energetic, and their behavior is just a manifestation of the discomfort they're feeling. Instead of punishment and shouting that only frighten and intimidate the child into submission, a parent can choose to deal with the situation by engaging and attending to them, perhaps taking them to the park to burn off some steam, or settling them down with a cuddle and something to eat before talking to them calmly about their behavior and helping them to see how their actions weren't acceptable and were a poor way to handle how they feel.

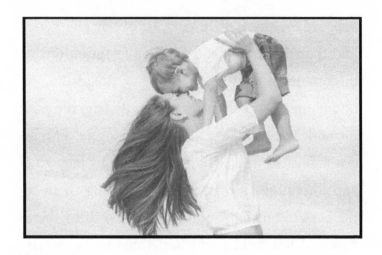

A lot of parents are skeptical of this approach at first. They tend to think it's too soft, and will result in badly behaved and spoiled kids. They're looking to correct bad behavior, and they associate behavior correction with raised voices and tears. Children can drive us up to the wall sometimes, so it's only right for people to want positive parenting to present them with a real solution to bad behavior. We've all been there. You spend a long, hard day at work, only to return home to a mess of a house. There's a thick atmosphere of tension. Your children have been misbehaving and resisting all attempts to control their behavior from your partner. This leads to you becoming frustrated and angry — you don't need this right now, not after the day you've had. You desperately want your children to just be well-behaved, happy, and easy to live with, and you don't understand why this isn't the case. Perhaps you find yourself wondering why your children are acting up, questioning whether you're doing something wrong or comparing your kids to other, well-behaved children and guiltily wishing yours were different.

This whole situation stems from a lack of true understanding between you and your children. They don't understand how much you're affected by the circumstances of your work life, or how hard it is to come home to a stressful environment. They don't understand why their behavior is so difficult, or why they're making your life harder. You don't understand how they can't see these things when it's all so obvious to you. The thing is, children see the world a very different way to us. They have little idea about the level of stress an adult has to deal with on a daily basis. They don't know how many things you're responsible for, how much pressure there is on you as a worker and a parent. The best way to rectify bad behavior is to help your children better understand you and how their behavior affects you to make them *want* to behave well, to develop their empathy. In the same way, if you can come to understand exactly why they're doing what they're doing, you can respond to instances of negative behavior in a much more effective way.

Forging a deeper understanding with your children isn't possible through becoming frustrated and shouting at them to behave. It takes a lot of patience and a deeper level of awareness of all the issues and factors at play in the situation in order to break it down and reach your children in a gentler way, a way that appeals to them way more than just being shouted at until they fall in line. Positive parenting cultivates a much calmer, less stressful home life through fostering this deeper understanding and connection between you and your kids. Sitting them down whenever they misbehave and softly explaining to them how it affects you and how hard it can make your life will over time enable you to reach them, to help them see how their behavior impacts other people and spark empathy within them. This will help them to put themselves in other people's shoes and be more considerate of how their actions affect those around them. This leads to more consideration from your children and from you, resulting in a far more laid back and easygoing atmosphere around the house.

A positive approach to parenting helps to encourage a sense of deep respect and cooperation between parents and their children. When everyone involved in an immediate family understands that there is no 'me vs. you', no power struggle, but instead only mutual love and respect amongst the team that is the family unit, problems suddenly become far easier to deal with. Genuinely connecting with children becomes possible and helping them to see things from a different point of view means you can reach them and make a real change where it's most needed.

A great example of this is when a child doesn't understand why what they've done is wrong — for example, if they wander off at the grocery store. A parent is obviously going to be extremely concerned and panicked by a situation like this, but a child might not really understand why. When we understandably react with panic and fear by shouting at them and ordering them never to do that again, they're left scared and confused without ever even truly understanding the gravity of the situation. A positive parenting based approach to this scenario would be to instead calmly have a conversation with them, informing them that we live in a dangerous world and that there are people out there who abduct children. As a parent, our job is to protect our children. If we don't know where they are, we can't protect them, so they should never wander off out of our sight in a public place because anything could happen and we wouldn't be able to stop it. Taking this approach does the same thing as simply shouting and controlling their behavior through fear, but in a very different way. It educates and informs your child, helping them to see why we have rules that they need to follow and allowing them to understand that we set these rules for their own best interests.

Once you set a healthy and mutually respectful tone with your children, they will appreciate it, even if it takes time for this appreciation to manifest itself in their behavior or words. Dealing with just a couple of issues in a positive way enhances the mood of everyone involved, and you'll soon see the difference it makes. Kids feel better; they feel enlightened. They understand you, themselves, and the reality of the situation of life more clearly, and they're very likely to want to go on using that approach in the future because it leaves them feeling like real progress has been made.

Positive parenting offers a number of benefits. Here are some of the following benefits:

- A calm, stress-free family atmosphere
- A loving emotional bond between parents and children
- Children feel affirmed and included

- Children have higher self-esteem
- Higher school grades
- Fewer behavior problems
- Lower rates of substance abuse
- Better social skills and friendships
- Children and parents feel happier
- Children are more likely to listen to and respect their parents, including an inclination to follow their parents' advice and wishes
- Increased sensitivity and understanding between parents and children

The effectiveness of positive parenting is exceptional. Not only does it serve to address immediate short-term concerns like curbing misbehavior and promoting politeness and respect in children, it also allows them to develop along clear, wholesome principles and moral and behavioral tangents that set them up with a variety of positive traits for later life such as kindness, respect for others, patience, compassion, a desire for greater insight, a clearer understanding in all circumstances, emotional stability (a greater ability to process and regulate emotions), well-developed ethical and moral principles and considerations, and positive moods and states of mind. In short, positive parenting helps shape children into good, honest, responsible and ethical people.

In addition to this, positive parenting fosters close and loving relationships among the members of the family unit. It reduces stress, depression, and negative feelings and resentment to an astonishing extent. It improves the quality of life of parents and children alike, leading to an increased sense of wellbeing, peace, and happiness amongst all members of the family. The quality of someone's home life and childhood is a direct indicator of their future happiness, wellbeing, and success in life. Being raised in a way that incorporates aspects of positive parenting will massively enhance a person's potential to live a content and peaceful life full of love and laughter.

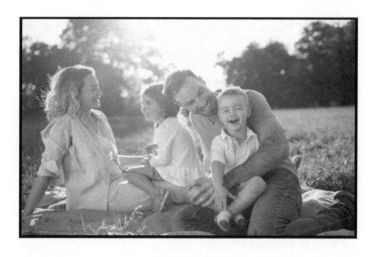

The increasingly popular trend of positive parenting is a revolutionary development in human history. In much the same way as liberating children from the factories of the early post-industrial revolution western world helped spur our society on to the level of development and opportunity that we possess today, positive parenting can help us to raise future generations in a way that encourages and builds them up to make the most out of life and treat others the way they were treated as kids, rather than leaving them feeling empty and disappointed with life like so many people are. The benefits of positive parenting are essentially endless, with virtually no drawbacks. There aren't any disadvantages to raising children in a positive and loving manner and making sure they feel well understood, cared for, and loved.

This outlook is what's really at the heart of positive parenting. It's about building healthier relationships between parents and our children. This approach helps parents to understand how to interact with our children in a more sensitive, self-aware, and consistent manner. This ensures that children are happier and more optimistic, which in turn strengthens the bond they have with their parents and makes them more likely to be respectful, well-behaved, thoughtful, and mindful of others. It encourages a feedback loop of mutual respect and understanding of each other as human beings, regardless of age, that helps us all to press on, grow, and develop in a deeply beneficial and beautiful way.

One of the great advantages of the Positive Parenting Theory is this emphasis on looking forward instead of backward. It's based on the idea that there's no such thing as a good or bad child, only good and bad behavior. The aim of positive parenting is to focus on correcting bad behavior and cultivating the good by focusing on what the reality of a situation is as it's happening and what can be changed and improved, rather than dwelling on the past or things that you wish were different but can't change. All too often, people find themselves stuck on certain events that have happened in the past that they hold a grudge over. This is anything but productive. All it does is cause resentment between parents and their children. Instead of punishing children for things that might have happened in the past, positive parenting theory focuses on learning and changing in the present for the future.

It's this focus on the future that really helps positive parenting to make such incredible headway when it comes to reaching children. It's strongly associated with greater wellbeing in later life; lower rates of substance abuse, better self-esteem, and a better ability to make friends are all huge indicators of future success for our children. If a child learns how to process and regulate their emotions and interact with themselves and the people around them in a healthy way, including being self-confident enough to resist peer pressure and make their own decisions, as well as understanding how to seek out and make friends with other like-minded individuals, they're equipped with an excellent tool kit for managing their lives and becoming responsible adults. They're more likely to be able to make responsible, decisions that take multiple factors into account, rather than acting impulsively and getting themselves into trouble.

The Role And Purpose
Of A Parent

Positive parenting involves considering your purpose as a parent and taking stock of the role you play in your children's lives. For some people, their position as a parent is a lifelong role. It is total and unconditional, lasting right until the day they die, in whatever capacity their children might need them. These parents would be happy for their children to live with them, even as adults. Others see their responsibility for their children's wellbeing extending only so far as keeping them alive and healthy until the day that they become an adult, and no further. Some parents will kick their children out of the home on their eighteenth birthday and leave them to fend for themselves. The very fact that you're reading this book right now suggests that you're in the former group. I'm not advocating infantilizing your children into adulthood — far from it — but positive parenting involves understanding the full nature and potential of your role as a parent. There is a wide gulf between your legal obligation as a parent and the level to which you can provide your child with a wealth of care and love to set them up as well as possible for later life.

You possess the ability to not only be a guardian for your children, but to be a teacher, mentor, guide, caretaker, and friend to them as well. The truth of the matter is that you can give as much of yourself to your children as you choose to. It's not a zero-sum game. Their gain is not your loss. On the contrary, the more of yourself that you give, the more of your time and energy and laughter and love you provide for your children, the more you will gain. In return, you will receive all of their time, their energy, their laughter, their love, and their care for you. Raising children is an extraordinarily rewarding and beautiful experience. You have the ability to shape young hearts and minds, to help them achieve their wildest dreams and support them through their darkest moments.

You are your children's primary role model. They interact with you every day, observe you, soak up your every word, every facial expression, every movement. Children learn by imitation; all this forms the basis, the template of their own personality that they will edit and sculpt into their own as they grow older. To your child, you are the sum total of almost their entire experience. Nearly every single thing they are conscious of, especially before they start going to preschool, is run through the filter of your presence. Through your behavior, they are given insight into how an adult is supposed to behave. They learn by observation and imitation and will use you as the barometer against which they compare all of their interactions with other adults. A good parent, therefore, makes all the difference for a child. Not only does the relationship they have with you shape their childhood, but it also reflects the life they will lead as an adult to a large extent.

You have the power to influence the type of life your children will lead, and therefore the life of their own children one day. Your actions create your family's legacy. The stamp you put on your children will follow them throughout the rest of their lives. It will impact the way they decide to bring up their children, for better or worse. Your decisions and actions directly correlate with the quality of life your children experience for the rest of their lives. Once your children have grown up, left the nest, and are busy living lives of their own, you will continue to play a significant part in their lives. You might not be responsible for their wellbeing anymore, but you will remain of central importance to them as their parent — one of the closest relationships you can have with another human being. Plenty of people have difficult and strained relationships with their parents as adults, which more often than not is at least in part the result of resentment left over from their childhood, from the feeling that the way in which they were raised was lacking and left them feeling afraid and insecure.

Positive parenting requires a great deal of reflection about your role as a parent, the relationship you want to have with your children, and the relationship you had with your own parents growing up. Incorporating positive parenting into the way in which you raise your children means completely embracing the multitude of roles you can potentially play for them. Next, I'll outline the main roles you can perform for your children throughout the different stages of their lives.

The Caretaker

The first and the most fundamental and important role you play for your children is as their caretaker. This involves keeping them safe, fed, happy, clothed, and providing access to education. This is a role that fluctuates in intensity throughout their life; a newborn requires far more caretaking than a teenager, and once your children have grown up and moved out, your time as a caretaker comes to an end. However, you might find that one day your children have kids of their own, and suddenly you're back to playing the role of caretaker again. This job cuts both ways, though. When you're elderly and need help taking care of yourself, your children will be there to care for you when you need them just like you were there for them.

Being a caretaker might not sound like the most glamorous job in the world, but it is a necessary one. Your primary job as a parent is to look after

41

your children, and that means getting stuck in and doing the hard, messy jobs. Even this, though, is an incredibly rewarding and beautiful experience. The look on your child's face when they're well fed, happy, and safely tucked up in bed at night as you read them a story and kiss them goodnight makes everything worth it.

The Guide, Mentor, and Teacher

As your children's guide, your role is to show them the ropes of how to be human. You teach them how to speak, you socialize them, you raise them with an understanding of what is required of them in the culture in which they are brought up. You show them the way in life and teach them how to survive. You train them to use the bathroom and feed themselves, help them with their homework, and give them guidance when they go to school and begin to encounter the complexities of socializing with strangers and making friends. In this role, you are responsible for their mental, emotional, and social development. You are a living, breathing role model for your children, and through you, they learn about the world around them.

Performing this role for your children is by far the most enlightening part of being a parent. You get to see in real time how your influence rubs off on your kids, how they adopt your mannerisms and speech and ways of handling situations. The biggest part of playing this role isn't setting out to teach your children anything directly but simply helping to mold and shape them through your everyday presence in their lives and by demonstrating how you act and react to certain situations. Once your children are fully grown, you continue to play this part in their lives, even though you now find yourself on an equal footing. Children are capable of teaching you lessons about the world and life in exactly the same way you teach them. I know that I've had my breath taken away countless times by the insightful comments my children have said, and the unique and beautiful ways of thinking and looking at the world that they've shown me. Once they're fully grown, your kids are able to assist you in this role, as well. They will have their own mature, well-developed outlooks on life, their own attitudes, their own experiences of the world that can help to shape you in exactly the same way you shaped them. Parenting is an interactive, reciprocal experience; both you and your children will change because of each other's influence throughout the course of your lives.

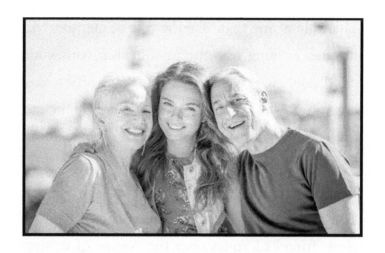

The Friend

Perhaps the most under-appreciated role you will play for your children — particularly when they're teenagers — is that of one of their closest and most trusted friends and confidants. You play with them, talk to them, answer their questions about the world, read to them, and spend time in their company. You take them on days out, organize their birthday parties, entertain them, and introduce them to virtually every new part of the world that they experience.

This role is one that, like the role of mentor, will last for as long as your relationship with your child does. It's one that changes and progresses over time as you and your child come to understand ourselves and each other more completely.

You may not feel like your child is a particularly close friend of yours over the course of raising them, and that's okay. It's perfectly normal to feel that way. Part of your duty to your child is to understand that they may not always appreciate or value all of the things you do for them and how much you care about their wellbeing. The fact of the matter is, you will always be their mom or dad. When everything breaks down and they feel lost and abandoned, you will be their first port of call. You will be the person they rely on, the person they know they can count on to help pick them up and get them through a rough patch. That's because as their parent you're their oldest, closest friend, and you always will be whether they realize it right now or not.

Embracing Your Role as a Parent

One of the most important lessons of positive parenting is that you should throw yourself into every aspect of parenthood with total enthusiasm. You won't always succeed in living up to the expectations you have of yourself, the idea of the kind of parent you want to be, but that's normal; you're only human. Getting it right every time isn't possible or necessary. What is important is being able to completely embrace the role you have as a parent and being committed to trying over and over again until you get it right. This means getting back up every time you're knocked down, no matter how many times it happens. It means holding yourself responsible for your own words and actions and doing your utmost to better yourself and set a good example for your children whenever you can.

Being a good parent is about being a good human being. It's about your heart always being in the right place, regardless of whether things turn out how you were expecting them to or not. Throw yourself into parenting. Let yourself get involved in every aspect. Allow yourself to try and learn from the experiences you have no matter whether you fail or succeed. Be there for your kids. Take the time to get to know them, to learn what makes them tick. Listen to them when they talk to you about their thoughts, their feelings, their hopes, and dreams. And if you ever find yourself feeling guilty and remorseful for things, you could or should have done, forgive yourself. Accept that you're only human. Understand that the most important part of life is learning from your mistakes when you make them. Beating yourself up and wallowing in misery over situations that you can no longer change and actions you can't undo achieves anything. Look back only as much as you need to in order to learn from your mistakes and then go forward.

Being a parent is one of the most challenging things it's possible to do in life, so accept the challenge. Don't shrink from it. Don't let your fears about what could go wrong stop you from stepping up to the plate and taking your very best swing.

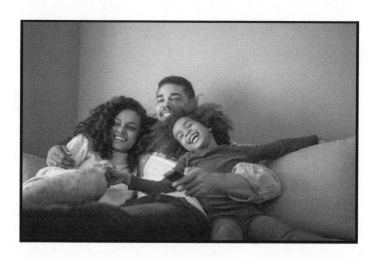

Hit or miss, it's the trying that matters. The more mistakes you make, the more you learn. The more you learn, the better a parent you become. Believe in yourself and in your capacity to be everything a child could ever want in their parent, and you'll find that you take to the role like a duck to water. The importance of having faith in yourself as a parent cannot be overstated. You have to have the courage to make difficult decisions and stick to them, to do what you think is best — not because you should always be right, but because if you're always second-guessing yourself you'll never make any progress. Embrace the beautiful journey that is parenthood.

Parental Cohesiveness

In order for positive parenting to be properly implemented, the entire parental unit in the family home has to be on board and willing to proceed with and stick to the methodology that will be outlined in this book. This means that you and your co-parent if you have one, need to maintain a united front in terms of your approach. You need to be consistent in your attitude to parenting your children at all times. If one of you is trying their best to positive parent while the other repeatedly lose their temper and handles situations badly, your children will become confused and unsure as to where they stand or how they should behave. This can lead to insecurity and feelings of self-doubt as they struggle to comprehend exactly what is and isn't acceptable for them to do and how their behavior will be interpreted and responded to by their parents.

That isn't to say you can't disagree with your partner in front of your kids, of course. In fact, if you can disagree in a healthy and mature way, staying level-headed and using calm reasoning to express your thoughts and feelings to each other in such a way that you gain a better understanding of each other's viewpoints in a positive manner, then letting your children see this healthy way of resolving disputes will be a boon to their personal development. Screaming and shouting at each other in front of your children, however, is never a good idea and can significantly upset them and teach them all of the wrong lessons about how to speak to the people they love.

The unique circumstances of your family situation will influence the options and tools that you have available to you as a parent. If you're a single parent or you're co-parenting with someone whom you're not in an active romantic relationship with, the situations you'll need to handle and the way in which you handle them will be different to those that you would face if you had a partner that you were parenting with. We'll go into detail regarding a few common types of parenting situation, the complications that arise from each, and how you can address them effectively no matter your individual situation.

Parenting as a Couple

The traditional western nuclear family consists of two parents and their children, with the parents either married or cohabiting and maintaining an intimate relationship with one another in addition to raising children together. Any type of co-parenting requires teamwork, of course, but this particular situation involves two people that in addition to working together solely to bring up a child, also have to work together to maintain their own romantic relationship with each other. This additional dynamic within the family unit can both complicate the act of bringing up kids and make it easier, depending on the relationship a particular parental couple has with each other.

The way in which parenting as a couple influences the development of the children in a family varies widely between different couples, but there are a few key areas which are affected by this particular parenting situation:

Setting a good example - As your children's main relationship model, the dynamic you share with your significant other will be internalized by your children and used as the bar against which they measure all of their future romantic relationships. If your relationship is lacking in any core values such as trust, respect, honesty, or effort, or the interaction you have with your significant other is underscored by aggression or maliciousness, your kids will pick up on it and consider it normal, because they have little insight into how an intimate relationship is supposed to be. Setting a bad example of a relationship for your children could have countless repercussions for them later on in life by giving them warped ideas of what is acceptable within the context of a relationship.

Arguments and Disputes - Any arguments and disputes you have with your partner will have an impact on your children. If you handle them poorly, with raised voices and insults, instead of sitting down and calmly talking through disputes, your children will pick up on this negativity and lack of respect between the two of you. It will demonstrate to them that the proper way to handle disagreement is to shout and scream and throw your weight around, rather than handling things maturely and with patience and understanding.

Unified authority - You and your partner represent the two main points of authority in your family. If you can be divided, you can be played against each other and conquered. Disagreements are fine, but when you make decisions, a unified stance has to be adopted. You have to parent as a team. If you're out shopping and your child wants to buy a new toy that you know you can't afford but your partner says yes, there's a problem. Suddenly, you're the bad guy in your child's eyes, even though you might be making the correct call. You have to make decisions together and naturally defer to one another. If you can cooperate and compromise, you can present a unified and consistent front to your children.

Communication - It's essential that both you and your partner communicate properly. If either of you needs to make a non-trivial decision, it's best to consult the other first, otherwise, you run the risk of a disagreement that forces you to backpedal, and the unified front breaks down. You also need to be up to date when it comes to things like your children's recent behavior or issues they've been struggling with so that you're both properly equipped to deal with them.

Differing attitudes - Both parents need to be on the same page in order to properly practice positive parenting. If either yourself or your partner isn't committed to the process, the result will be persistent and corrosive inconsistency in your actions and reactions that will only confuse your children and cultivate distrust and suspicion. If your children don't know that they can expect consistent reactions and advice from both of their parents, they will be more inclined to lie about things to avoid conflict and getting in trouble, and less likely to be honest with you. If one of their parents has a different, less empathetic and understanding attitude towards parenting, your children will find themselves picking favorites and tailoring their behavior to best suit whichever parent is around, which inevitably leads to a rabbit hole of further issues between both yourself and your partner and the relationship you have with your kids.

When you're trying to implement positive parenting as a couple you have to take these factors into account. You'll have a difficult time trying to raise your children in a positive manner if one of the most fundamental aspects of your family, the core relationship that it stems from and revolves around, isn't positive in itself. Parenting as a couple introduces new challenges stemming from your relationship that are up to you to identify and approach in the same way you'd approach issues with your children. The key thing here is to ensure that your relationship and your children alike are treated with as much respect, understanding, and patience as possible. You have to make an effort to ensure your relationship with your partner is solid and committed, and isn't neglected as a result of the immense strain that raising children can often inflict. Any issues within the relationship between yourself and your partner need to be acted upon quickly in order to prevent resentment from festering and eroding the bond you share together from within. Having children puts an immense amount of pressure on the relationship of the parents that are raising them, but whether you allow this pressure to overwhelm both of you or bring you closer together is up to you and your partner.

Co-parenting Outside of a Relationship

An increasingly large number of people these days are taking on a form of co-parenting, or parenting cooperatively, without being in a romantic relationship with the person they're parenting with. This can refer to any number of parental circumstances; ex-partners that have had kids before splitting up but continue to share the responsibility of raising them, grandparents that help their child raise their own children because otherwise, they'd be a single parent, adult offspring that help their parent bring up their siblings when there's a significant age gap, separated parents with partners of their own that also get involved (or step-parents), and so on and so forth. This type of parental situation is both similar to and yet differs significantly from one that stems from a romantic relationship; the parenting duties are shared amongst two (or

understanding support network that children so desperately need.

Another factor that must be taken into account is ensuring that your children feel adequately valued and wanted by everyone involved in raising them, particularly if they're being shuttled between each of their parent's homes on a weekly basis. Children in this situation are often left with the distinct impression that they're unwanted by one or more of their parents, particularly if they're seen as a burden or if there's a step-parent or step-family on the scene who — intentionally or not — make them feel like things have changed and they're no longer as important to the people raising them as they once were. Children are sensitive and can easily be wounded by perceived slights, regardless of how minor or unintentional they might be. They can't help this, of course. They lack the emotional and mental development and life experience to really put things in context and see issues from other points of view. All they know is that they feel upset and unprioritized, and once resentment has taken root it can fester and grow and become extremely difficult to overcome.

Children can have lasting scars from situations where they feel unloved or unwanted which continue to follow and haunt them far into their adult lives. Where issues like their parents splitting up are concerned, the uncertainty and insecurity they feel are amplified tenfold. Something as simple as one of their parents moving out and getting a dog can lead to them feeling like they've been replaced like their parent is now free of them and has decided to invest their time and energy into something else instead.

Particularly unconventional types of co-parenting, such as a child's grandparents directly helping to raise them, can cause further issues in a child's development that need to be addressed. Grandparents might not be as clued into the reality of the world the young generation face today, especially with regard to the role of social media and the internet. It's therefore essential that if this is the parenting situation that you're involved in you take an active interest in both the day to day life of your child and the unique issues they face so that you have a better idea of how to handle things when problems come up.

Single Parenting

A single parent is someone who represents the whole of the parental unit, even if they receive help with childcare from other family members. If you are the sole person with a direct and everyday parental relationship with your children, you're a single parent. This situation comes with a whole host of its own unique issues which have to be addressed fully in order to properly and effectively practice positive parenting. Being a single parent does come with advantages, however. For one thing, it's just you, so there's no need to worry about being unified in your approach or any of the other dynamics that come into play when you're parenting as a co-operative venture. Some of the issues you do need to take into account are:

Discipline - This can be an especially difficult problem for single mothers of boys, particularly if they're being influenced by other people (such as other boys at school) and are acting out, being aggressive and shutting down any attempts at helping them to rectify their behavior or highlighting to them that the way they're acting isn't acceptable. In an ideal world, practicing positive parenting right from the start should, for the most part, prevent problems of this nature, but this is only possible if you know about the theory of positive parenting right from the word go. Remember, all you can do is your best with the information you have at any one time. In addition to this, people are complicated and children of all ages can be heavily influenced by their peers and difficult or traumatic experiences can lead to inappropriate behavior regardless of your attempts to steer them in the right direction. Being a single parent makes discipline and behavior correction harder to implement because you don't have the emotional and practical support of a partner there with you to make sure the rules are enforced. If one of your kids is acting up and flat out refuses to do as they're told, you might feel flat-footed or that they've called your bluff. The presence of a partner here would solidify your position and allow you to stand firm and ensure your child faces consequences for their actions in order to help them learn what they can and can't do. Additionally, the presence of another parent provides more flexible options for calming children down, talking to them, and explaining the other parent's point of view when there has been a disagreement. Handling discipline as a single parent is notoriously tricky. You need to be prepared to have your own back and to stand your ground and be firm in your decisions. Having a strong support network of family and friends who know your child well and can help step in when they need to and express their disappointment in a gentle manner to try and reach your child will also go a long way towards effectively disciplining your children. Often, disappointment from someone your child respects is a far better motivator than anger.

Financial burden - Being a single parent often comes with a lot of financial difficulties. Providing for a family on a single income is hard, particularly if you're not receiving child support. There's no easy way out of this kind of situation. Planning and budgeting are your best friends here. You need to find a balance that works for you so that your children don't go without while also making sure they have a roof over their heads and food on the table. You should also take every precaution to make sure you don't make a difficult situation worse by having more children when you're still in a bad financial position.

Gender-specific issues - Single parents with children of the opposite sex can often struggle because they find it hard to relate to some situations that is largely gender-specific, such as a single father with a daughter beginning to go through puberty, or a single mother struggling to relate to her teenage son. As a parent, it's your job to dive headfirst into uncomfortable and difficult issues and do your very best to support and guide your children no matter how little you know about or relate to a particular situation. Educate yourself by reading books on the matter or watching videos online to get a better understanding of both the issues your child is facing and the mindset they are likely to have in order to better encourage and mentor them.

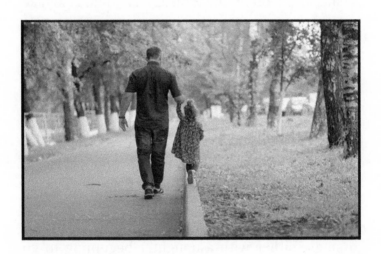

The Importance of Good Role Models

An extremely important aspect of a child's development is the presence of good role models. This is someone that the child can look up to and imitate the behavior of. Children learn primarily through observation and imitation, so this is a crucial part of their growth. A child should have someone of their own gender in their life that sets a good example for them in terms of how they think, talk, and behave, whose footsteps they can follow in and whose positive path in life they can emulate. In the modern era, unconventional families are becoming increasingly common, meaning more and more children are finding themselves without someone close to them who they really identify with and admire. This is an especially prominent concern when it comes to single parenting.

There's been a trend in recent years as the result of the increasing acceptance in society of non-conventional parental combinations such as homosexual or transgender parent couples, as well as raising children without putting pressure on them to conform to any kind of gender expectations. None of this is harmful to children's development — kids will grow up just fine regardless of whether they have a mother and father, two parents of the same sex, or a parent that's transgender. However, these situations (like any parenting situations) raise unique issues of their own. For example, if two male parents are raising a daughter, they should take care to ensure that she has the presence of a positive female role model in her life, in order to provide her with someone who she strongly identifies with and can offer her insight into what kind of person she wants to become. The best strategy is to give your child as many options as you can to let them decide their own preferences and identity as they grow up.

Without a strong role model, children can find it difficult to make their way in the world. They might feel lost or directionless, and can easily fall in with the wrong crowd who often provide them with the older role models they seek, people that they admire and feel they can look up to and imitate the behavior of. This is the sort of process that can lead to young boys falling in with hardened criminals and gang members who offer them a feeling of belonging, comradeship, and direction that they otherwise lack in their life. If you make sure that your children have the right kind of role models and direction, they will go a long way in life. Children are like sponges; they soak up the things they're exposed to and internalize them in order to survive in whichever circumstances they're brought up in. If you ensure your child is surrounded by positive and uplifting people and experiences, they'll be on the right path from an early age.

Exercise: The Positive Parenting Theory

1. Reflect

Now that you've come to the end of the first chapter of this handbook, allow yourself to pause and reflect on what you've read so far. Take as long as you need to process the positive parenting theory, the way in which it approaches the act of parenting and how it applies to your own role as a parent. Take a few deep breaths and try to center yourself into a calm and relaxed mindset, regardless of the difficulties in your life right now. There's nothing you can't try your best to handle, and at the end of the day, all you can do is your best.

It's a good idea to get some paper and a pen and jot down a few notes on whatever things are whirring about in your mind after having finished this chapter. How do you feel about the idea of parenting positively? How does it relate to your own experiences as a parent and as a child being brought up by your own parents? What kind of parent can you be for your children, how can you help them to become the best versions of themselves and have brilliant and fulfilling lives of their own?

2. Don't just look; see

The human mind is brilliant at zeroing in on and paying attention to one thing at a time. This allows us to drink in all of the details of what we're focusing on. However, it can also make it hard for us to see the bigger picture. Sometimes it can be hard to see the forest because you're focusing on the trees. Learning to really see the full context of any situation involves stepping back and looking at how different factors fit together and combine to form a complex series of interacting parts that influence and depend upon each other. Think of it like a jigsaw puzzle. You can't just look at each individual piece one at a time, one after the other, and hope to complete it. You have to step back and see it all laid out in order to try and see how it's all pieced together. Parenting is very much a process of stepping back and seeing the bigger picture, so practicing this skill will help you to no end.

Imagine that you are feeling overwhelmed and you confront a situation that makes you want to scream at the top of your lungs. Perhaps you've just spent money decorating your child's bedroom, only to walk in and find that they've drawn on the walls with a marker pen. Responding to this very upsetting and stressful scenario in a positive and constructive way involves stepping back from the scene mentally and taking inventory of how all the little pieces are put together in order to assess your internal mindset at that moment. You've put in the time, effort, and hard-earned money in order to create a nice environment for your child, and in just a few moments they've managed to ruin it. You are understandably upset, so your natural reaction will probably be one of anger and disappointment. Looking at the bigger picture here means understanding your own mental state and why you feel the way you feel, and then putting yourself in your child's shoes. They lack the level of emotional and mental development necessary in order to fully comprehend what they've done — drawing on the walls was an innocent act of creativity, not an attempt to spite you or ruin all of the hard work you put in.

Being able to see this fully at the moment (or afterwards upon reflection, if this isn't immediately possible) will allow you to swallow your rage and handle the situation in a more understanding and productive way. Rather than getting angry and shouting at the child, you could calmly explain that you spent a lot of time and money on decorating their room and that by drawing on the walls they've hurt your feelings and potentially cost you more time and money for redecoration. This will have a far more effective outcome in terms of helping the child to understand why what they have done is unacceptable and correct this behavior in order to avoid it in the future than simply shouting at them would, while simultaneously avoiding the negative, stressful, and upsetting experience (for both you and them) of telling them off. When we reach a volatile emotional state, we're like a volcano that's ready to blow. It's easier to explode and go ballistic than it is to keep a cool head and address the situation with a thought-out approach, but it becomes easier with practice. If you don't succeed in keeping your cool in a situation like this, don't beat yourself up about it. You're only human, and this is a

difficult skill to master. Just keep at it and you'll
see results.

Part Two:

Positive Parenting In Action

Communication is one of those elusive and slippery concepts that most people understand is important in theory but few really grasp the true significance and potential of.

Communication And Conflict

As human beings, we're extremely social animals. In fact, we're the most social animals on earth. Our ability to work together as a team has allowed us to evolve, survive, and progress to the position we hold now, with a dominant global civilization that influences every aspect of the natural world around us, for better or worse. Communication has been key to our development. It is the defining trait of being human. Without the ability to communicate, we would lack the basic requirements to begin even constructing complex thoughts and ideas, because we couldn't even begin to communicate what we knew to ourselves and therefore build upon our own foundations of knowledge.

Luckily, we can all be taught to communicate. But communication is a deeply complicated thing that stretches far beyond simple teamwork and problem solving as a group. Communication is a skill and one that begins to resemble a superpower when it's developed to a significant extent. Take this book, for example. Through written communication, I can provide you with abstract and complex information that you can take in, process, and then apply in your own life to your own and your family's immediate benefit; that's only one example of the limitless potential of communication.

There are two specific desires that virtually every person on this earth craves and needs, whether they're aware of it or not. To be loved, and to be understood. Each of us exists in our own private world of infinite complexity and difficulty. As human beings, we're both incredibly similar to one another and excruciatingly unique at the exact same time. The extent to which we can communicate is the extent to which we can give others an insight into the individual universe that each of us possesses and exists inside of on an everyday basis. If we can communicate well, we can allow others a glimpse of insight into the inner workings of our minds and help them to understand us that bit better. It is impossible for any one person to ever be completely understood, as in order to totally understand another person we would have to be that person; we'd have to go through each of the unique experiences of that person's life that shaped their mindstate into the form it exists in today.

Communication is the ether through which we develop our relationships with others and with ourselves. When we communicate effectively, we break down the barriers that divide each of us and cultivate stronger, more empathetic, more aware and understanding bonds with others. Communication, then, is the single most effective tool you possess in your relationships with your children. Developing and sustaining great communication channels with your children leads to a two-way street of enhanced understanding between you and them, helping you to shape and guide them in a positive way. Having open, honest, mature conversations with your children is essential to positive parenting.

How to Communicate Well

When it comes to learning how to communicate well with your children, the essential thing that you need to understand is that saying the right thing in the right way is only half of the process — and it's arguably the less important part. Listening is the key to good, revealing conversation. The art of listening, much like the art of talking, can be a difficult skill to practice. Although both listening and talking can be challenging things to learn how to do well, most people find it far easier to talk than to listen. If you've ever had a conversation with someone where you see their eyes glaze over as they stop attention to you and start thinking about what they're going to say when it's their turn to speak, you'll know what I mean. The reason that this is so common is that talking is an active activity, whereas listening is passive. Active skills are easier to practice. They're rewarding; they make us feel like we're doing something because we're expressing ourselves and getting some of that infinite internal potential out there into the world. Talking can be immensely satisfying and relieving. If you have something that's weighing heavily on your mind, then opening up and confiding in someone can lift the pressure off of your shoulders almost instantly.

Passive activities like listening, though, don't have this intrinsically rewarding aspect to them. That's not to say that listening isn't rewarding, however. In fact, in my opinion, it is one of the most rewarding things it's possible for a person to do. The rewarding nature of listening is more difficult to access, however. It involves processing the words of another person and seeing the joy that can be found in learning more about them, in coming to understand them more deeply, and also in seeing the wisdom and value in the things they say and learning to understand yourself better as a direct result of this. Listening really isn't as hard as people make it out to be. Just pay attention to what another person says, and reflect on the words they use and their meaning. When your child talks, listen to them. Resist the urge to talk unless it's to further probe or encourage them to reveal their thoughts and feelings. If you can get into the habit of listening to your children more intently, you'll find that the understanding of each other the two of you share grows ever-deeper.

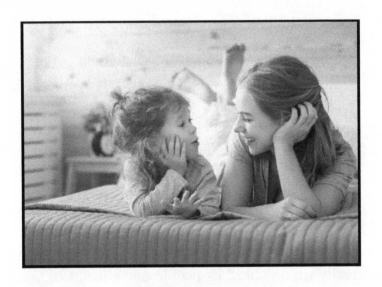

In order to communicate well, listen carefully and ask questions that are aimed at provoking a long answer from the person you're talking to. Communication is an interactive experience, so you'll get your opportunity to talk as well. When you do, address the things that were said by the other person. Offer them your thoughts on what they said, provide your own opinion, and ask further questions to better understand what they're trying to tell you. If, for example, your child is talking to you about their day at school, then participate completely in the experience of talking about school, purely for the sake of doing so. Pay attention to the little details and let yourself be curious about building up a clearer picture of the world your child experiences every day. If they tell you about something their teacher said, you could ask them what they thought about that. You could ask them what their fellow students think about things. The potential there is for learning about another person's experience as a human being is infinite, and you are limited only by your own interest. If you can cultivate a strong interest in your children's lives, you can establish a deeper, more meaningful relationship with them, built on a solid bedrock of good communication.

Healthy Communication

There are a lot of parents who become frustrated by their children talking too much. They yell at them to be quiet because they find them annoying, or they're trying to concentrate on something else. We all get frustrated from time to time, but these are examples of unhealthy communication that will lead to problems further down the line because a child on the receiving end of this kind of behavior feels invalidated and unloved. They feel as though their parents don't care about them or what they have to say. They feel insignificant, irrelevant, and small. These impressions can imprint into their psyche and follow them for the rest of their life, influencing their future relationships and happiness in a very negative way.

As I've already mentioned, communication is a two-way street. Healthy communication requires a lot of giving and taking. You have to take the time to listen to your children and make them feel validated in order to show them that their opinion has been heard and is valued by everyone in the family. Your children should be allowed to speak their minds, have their voices heard, and contribute those things they feel they can to the lives of the other members of their family. A great way to do this is to have family meals every day where the whole family has the opportunity to talk and listen to each other and everyone can feel heard. Additionally, take the time to speak to each of your children one-on-one on a regular basis to develop the personal connection you share with them.

You can't focus all of your attention on them constantly, of course. You have things to do, and children tend to not stop talking about anything and everything on account of them being relatively new to the world and therefore totally fascinated by virtually every new experience they have. Part of developing healthy communication is to learn to balance your time and help your child to understand this balance. If your child recognizes that when you're busy you won't be able to talk to them as much, but that you'll make up for it by coming to chat when you're no longer busy, they'll feel much more secure in themselves and comfortable to simply do their own thing in the meantime, safe in the knowledge that they'll get the conversation and close interaction with you that they desire soon enough.

The most effective way to teach your children lessons is through healthy communication. Sitting them down on a regular basis and having good, long, deep, honest conversations is the best way to:

a) **Teach them to listen and communicate well**

b) **Impart guidance and advice**

When you take the time to have conversations like this with your kids, you're teaching them how to communicate in a healthy way by showing them how to talk and listen in a manner that is open and honest. Your patience and understanding will directly rub off on them and show them how to do the same thing in return for you. Having calm, loving conversations like this might feel out of place for some people, especially those that would expect to have this kind of relationship with other adults, rather than children. However, children understand far more in a much more profound way than older people often give them credit for. In addition to this, by treating them like the little people they are and practicing healthy conversation with them, you're showing them how to grow into a mature and responsible adult. Holding these types of conversations with your kids will mean that in time they become better at having them and look forward to them immensely. Everyone wants to be understood, and these conversations represent a great opportunity for this to take place. You'll also be laying the groundwork for opportunities to impart your wisdom and guidance to your child in a way that they can fully understand and appreciate.

The Advantages of Good Communication

Establishing a good standard of dialogue with your child opens up an unlimited number of doors and presents endless possibilities for their personal growth and development. Just a few of the many benefits for your child of good communication include:

- An enhanced level of self-reflection
- A heightened sense of responsibility
- A mild-mannered, reasonable nature
- Politeness and patience

- Increased maturity
- A greater understanding of the world and their place within it
- Improved consideration of and a keener sense of respect for others and themselves
- An honest, open nature
- An introspective and inquisitive outlook
- Better self-esteem
- A well-developed and regulated emotional intelligence
- Enhanced decision-making capabilities

The art of communication can be incredibly effective in shaping a child into a young person that possesses and displays all of these attributes as a matter of their being. These are the kind of principles that are internalized and stick with a person as they expand their understanding of the world and the way things are. They are the core moral and ethical framework around which a young person can continue to develop and grow as they blossom into a balanced, confident, secure, and happy adult, even as they pass through the trials and tribulations that come with ascending into adulthood.

Developing a sturdy and level foundation for a child in this way becomes a boon throughout the rest of their life. It forms a pattern, a way of looking at the world and themselves, that they can use to tackle and overcome any obstacles that they come across throughout the length and breadth of their time on earth. As they continue to learn and grow from the lessons they learn as a result of handling tough situations with a positive and reflective mindset, they will maintain and increase their understanding of themselves as a direct result of the great communication and bond they have with you.

The benefits that this process contains for a child's emotional development is especially influential for their future happiness and satisfaction. We're highly emotional beings; whether we admit it to ourselves or not, our emotions are the driving force behind the decisions we make and the paths we choose to take throughout our lives. People with poorly developed emotional intelligence tend to be far more unhappy and impulsive, with a lower quality of life and standard of living, a habit of dwelling on past mistakes and how much they lack rather than appreciating the good things in their life, an attraction to dramatic and confrontational situations, a 'victim' mindset that results in a reduced capacity to take responsibility for their own actions, and a reduced capability to develop strong and stable intimate relationships and friendships. Communication and the understanding of emotions are the keys to leading a happy and fulfilling life. If you can cultivate these qualities in your child, they have an excellent chance of living a successful, content, and peaceful life filled with love and laughter.

Handling Conflict

Communication is the key to effectively dealing with difficult situations. Conflict is as natural to us as it gets. We're intrinsically wired to be motivated to protect our own self-interests and by extension those of the people and things we care about. When we feel like these are under threat in some way, our instinctual response is to get scared and angry. This has ensured our survival for millennia in the wilderness; it's programmed into our DNA. Helping a child to overcome these intense feelings and deal with the conflict they will face throughout their lives as well as managing the presence of conflict within your own home and family and between you and your children all comes down to communication.

For some parents, the way to deal with conflict is punishment and anger, especially when it comes to their child fighting with them. Any conflict is seen as disrespectful at best and an attempt to upset the 'power balance' between parent and child at worst, and is therefore usually handled with screaming matches and slamming doors. The thing is, this tends to do little to resolve the underlying reasons for conflict and doesn't defuse a tense atmosphere. All it does is make things worse and breed resentment for everyone involved. Where there's smoke, there's fire, and where there's conflict, there's deep emotional pain. The best way to approach conflict, therefore, is to try and get at this underlying hurt in everyone involved and deal with it so that all parties can make up and move on without feelings of bitterness and resentment.

An important point to make here is that people will do what they must, to defend themselves and protect their egos from harm and humiliation, no matter how old they are. Your children might even scream and shout at you when they're extremely wound up. You have to try your hardest to avoid taking this personally. Of course, it's unacceptable behavior, but at the moment it's happening your child feels fully justified in what they're doing and don't particularly care if you don't agree. It's perfectly natural for them to react that way, so rather than charging into butt heads with them, take a more careful and considered approach to things.

Whenever conflict kicks off, the first thing that needs to happen is to separate anyone involved and give them time to cool off, potentially including yourself. When people are angry and upset, they're highly emotionally charged. They lack the ability to properly think things through. They don't want to think things through. They want to scream and break things, and that's exactly what they'll do if you attempt to resolve the conflict then and there. Nothing productive is going to happen while they're still in that mindstate. Once everyone involved has calmed down, you can approach them individually and try to talk things out. You need to get to the bottom of why the conflict occurred and get all of the facts straight. If your child is obviously angry and upset and won't tell you why, try your best to avoid becoming frustrated with them, because that will only make the problem worse. They'll only shut down and block you out further because they're not receiving the love and support they so desperately need when they're facing difficult circumstances in their life, whether these happen to be internal or external in origin.

It's wise to keep in mind that the root causes of conflict are often very difficult for an outside observer to perceive. A person might be in deep emotional pain, feeling the pressure every day of their lives, and only give us any sign that they're in trouble when we see the pain manifested in their behavior when they snap at us or lash out in some way. An example of this could be your child being bullied at school, and doing their utmost to keep it secret from anyone but finding themselves easily frustrated and short-tempered. This could lead to outbursts of bad behavior, which may seem to you to have no discernible cause. We, therefore, have to keep an open mind when our children are hurting and won't tell us why and do our best to be there for them and remind them that we're here to help whenever they feel ready to talk to us.

You should understand that your child will sometimes need time to process what they're going through to the point where they feel able to talk to you about it. In the meantime, give them all of the love, encouragement, understanding, and space that you can in order to reduce the pressure they feel. When you do this, you'll find that they often come to you on their own terms to open up and ask for advice. Before someone can open up, they have to be able to feel comfortable enough to do so. Your job is to cultivate an atmosphere where they feel they can do this, not crack their shell by brute force and make them talk to you about what's going on.

When you do finally have an opportunity to talk to the people involved in any conflict properly, whether it's not long afterward or it takes a few days or weeks, there are two things that you need to address. The first is to discuss any underlying issues or grievances that led to the conflict, working out where they stem from, and then working on how to sort them out; the second is to make it clear that no matter what someone is feeling, conflict isn't the way to deal with those emotions. Outbursts of anger, violence, raised voices, abuse — none of it is productive. You should explain that negative emotions make us feel powerful and cause us to more easily lose control of our behavior, as though we were watching it happen to someone else, rather than ourselves. The way to approach these things is to help your child understand that it's okay to feel those negative emotions. Make it clear that the best way to react to these feelings, however, is to simply let them be there. Underline that your child shouldn't attempt to push them away or let them control them. If they can simply accept that they're there and that that's okay, no matter how difficult they are to experience, they can make sure that their negative feelings don't overpower them. Tell them that it's a good idea to remove themselves from any situation that has the potential for conflict as soon as they need to in order to allow themselves to calm down and avoid making a bad situation worse.

When we're actively involved in a conflict where we're shouting and causing drama, we've allowed our emotions to get the best of us. We've lost control over our equanimity of mind. Our calm, peaceful daily reality has been wrenched away from us, whether it's with or without our permission. Preventing this from happening in the future involves learning to regulate our own emotions. That isn't to say that we should ignore them or pretend they don't bother us, but rather attend to them as soon as we become aware of them and seek to learn more about them and why we're feeling them. The answer is always understanding. When you can understand the things you're feeling, you can control them better. You have power over them, rather than them having all of the power in influencing how you behave. You choose to indulge them or just let them slowly dissipate. Teaching your children how to regulate their emotions will help them move forward in life with a far better toolkit for handling intense and emotionally difficult situations, preventing frequent conflict from arising and allowing things to be talked out in a calm and peaceful way when it does.

Emphasize to your children that we can learn to feel a sense of detachment from our thoughts and feelings. They're part of us, but they don't have to define us. We don't have to immediately react to the thoughts that pop into our heads and the emotions that well up inside of us. We can simply allow them to be present and look at them with a sort of detached curiosity, as though they were happening to someone else. With this enhanced perspective, we can process the emotion in a calmer, more rational manner. Why are we feeling this way? What caused it? What do we want to do about it? What should we do about it? Taking this approach to the negative feelings we experience allows us to process them and deal with them in a healthy and constructive manner through understanding them first and then engaging with the second, rather than simply allowing ourselves to be swept away by them without a second thought as we might otherwise be prone to doing.

Dealing With the Conflict in Your Child's Life

For most well adjusted, stable, mature people, conflict isn't a part of everyday life. It is, however, a permanent feature of life itself, no matter the lengths you go to in order to avoid it. We all face conflict from time to time, and it's horrible every time. That's the reason why it's so essential that you properly prepare your child for the difficulties they'll face throughout the course of their lives. Making sure they understand how to process and regulate their emotional state is one thing, but teaching them how to handle the conflict they face, especially when it's other people who are upset and angry, is another entirely.

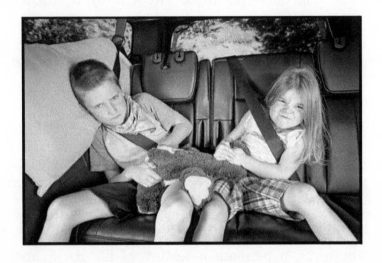

Conflict resolution is primarily about the attitude that we approach the circumstances of conflict that we're confronted with. Healthy conflict resolution consists of a state of mind that seeks to understand issues and grievances and defuse tension by talking things out, as opposed to just trying to deal with problems with aggression, shouting matches, insults, or violence. It's about understanding that dealing with problems in these kinds of ways only leads to them growing more complicated and out of control, which lessens our ability to deal with them. The best way to approach conflict is to try and be reasonable, careful, and decisive. Choose a carefully considered course of action and then take it. Try to teach your kids that most of the problems they'll face with other people can simply be talked out as long as they're smart about it. Choosing moments wisely in order to try and reach out and discuss issues with other conflicting parties in a relatively calm and peaceful atmosphere is important, which is why allowing for time to let the dust settle is usually a good idea. Once the dialogue is underway, it's important to be proactive in being open and apologizing for your own wrongdoing in order to encourage others to act in the same way.

However, not all conflict can be resolved in a peaceful way. Some people will not listen to reason and common sense. Some people are just looking for a fight, and this can be an issue for children young and old alike. Obviously, it's not a good idea to encourage physical violence or verbal abuse in any circumstances. Make it clear to your children that they should seek out authority figures like teachers or responsible adults in order to help defuse tense situations that could lead to physical confrontation. However, this isn't always possible either, and you have to reassure your child that you're behind them no matter what by letting them know that if they're in physical danger they should do whatever is appropriate and responsible to defend themselves in the form of fighting back. Again, physical violence should *always* be avoided wherever possible, but we live in a harsh world and not every child has the kind of parents that yours does. Avoiding conflict isn't always possible, so teach your child to stick up for themselves and protect themselves when they need to.

Some children will have more trouble than others at processing and regulating their feelings and behavior, especially when it comes to extremely powerful emotions like anger. If your child has a lot of difficulties controlling their anger, then it might be a good idea to see a professional anger management expert to get advice that's tailored to your child's specific circumstances. Being as understanding, encouraging, and loving as you can help your child to make progress for themselves, safe in the knowledge that their family is supporting them through the challenging process of learning to understand and manage their strongest emotions.

Apart from seeking outside help, some more things you can do to help your child to manage their anger better include:

Teaching them to differentiate between their feelings and behavior - you can help your child to better understand why they feel the way they feel and demonstrate to them that they don't have to respond to any situation in any particular way. Communicate to them that no matter how badly they might want to react to something in a certain way, they always have a choice. There is always the opportunity to pause, reflect, and choose not to respond to something, no matter how much it may seem like no choice exists.

Displaying your own anger management skills for them to observe and imitate - one of the best ways to teach your kids to manage their anger appropriately is to show them how it's done. Respond in a healthy and productive way when you're faced with difficult and frustrating scenarios to model positive ways of regulating anger and strong emotion for your children.

Showing them healthy ways to cope with overwhelming emotions - better methods of dealing with strong negative feelings include things like going for a walk, making a drink and taking a few minutes to calm down, laughing and joking about difficult situations with close friends and family (this is also known as dark humor), and taking out their anger in a physical way such as exercise or squeezing a stress ball. When we're angry, we have a lot of pent up energy that needs an outlet so this method can be especially effective at venting negative emotions.

Ensuring they understand that their actions have consequences and that aggressive behavior can't and won't just be tolerated - as much as we have to support our children and try to understand the difficulties they're facing in order to parent positively, we also have to make it clear to them that letting their anger manifests itself as violence or aggression is unacceptable, even if it can't be helped, and that it won't be tolerated. Angry outbursts must have consequences in order for a child to have a strong incentive to learn to control themselves. If they're able to be as angry and as destructive as they like without facing consequences, they will have little reason to try and improve themselves; they'll simply get used to getting away with it.

Bullying

This is a particularly important part of the world of conflict for us to examine. Bullying is a horribly common experience. Figures from *bullyingstatistics.org* suggest that up to 77% of students will experience some form of bullying throughout their school lives. But it's not just kids that are affected — bullying occurs right across the spectrum of the whole population. All kinds of people are the victims of bullying at all of the different stages of life. The fact that bullying is such a common and intimidating occurrence means that it's crucial to teach your children how to respond to it correctly so that if they encounter it in school or in the later part of their lives they're prepared to handle it.

Cambridge English dictionary defines a bully as 'someone who hurts or frightens someone else, often over a period of time, and often forcing them to do something that they do not want to do.' Bullying can be a subtle and highly subjective process, however, which is why it is so often masked behind humor to try and deflect and distract attention from the cruelty behind it. This is what is truly at the heart of bullying; using cruelty as a means of intimidating, exerting power and influence on, and controlling people.

Bullying can be a slippery concept because it can take many different forms, especially with the introduction of the internet in the modern area. It's hard to pin down exactly what bullying is. Some people hear the word and immediately conjure up mental images of playground jocks shaking down other kids for their lunch money and beating them up. For many people, if the police don't need to get involved because no laws have been broken, then bullying hasn't taken place — especially when it takes place at school, and can be shrugged off as harmless teasing and a natural part of growing up. The truth of bullying is that it's an extremely broad and circumstantial process. It might be natural, but it's never harmless. It can be an extremely damaging experience, even if no laws are broken, no money taken, and no blood is drawn. Bullying can involve something as simple as groups not letting individuals sit with them at lunch, or calling them names, spreading rumors, persuading neutral people not to talk to them, et cetera. Even this relatively basic level of bullying can be incredibly distressing and damaging for anyone to experience, but it's particularly hard for children, especially when it's more insidious, as it often is.

With the advent of social media and the place it now holds in our lives, much bullying occurs online, a phenomenon known as 'cyberbullying'. It's hard to overstate just how sickening and horrifying cyberbullying can be. These days, most kids on the playground have smartphones from a young age. This not only gives children the ability to record embarrassing or controversial situations but ensures that it's spread around the internet in minutes, meaning a very large number of people can become aware of and start to joke and gossip about these situations in a very short space of time. The viral nature of the online world means that these jokes and malicious gossip can spread like wildfire. It's not unheard of for a student to move schools because of bullying and find that everyone at their new school has already heard all about it once they get there. Nicknames and references to distressing and embarrassing situations can persist in a child's everyday life at school and then continue even once they're home where they should be safe and happy.

Cyberbullying can take nearly any form. It's limited only by the imagination of its perpetrators and can be targeted towards certain individual victims who are subject to persistent harassment, rumors, and gossip, which can even come from anonymous accounts that keep people's details hidden so the victim doesn't know exactly who it is that's tormenting them. In this way, something that started out as a slight problem can be exacerbated and grow into something that would be extremely difficult for anyone to cope with, let alone a young and impressionable child who can easily be convinced that their world is crumbling and their life is no longer worth living over something as trivial as embarrassing or incriminating screenshots that make them the center of a storm of drama.

The depersonalized and often anonymous nature of cyberbullying can make some kids easy targets for manipulation and blackmail. If, for example, someone threatens to spread a rumor or picture or video that someone would rather everyone they know didn't see (this can include extended family members on social media as well as just friends, heightening the intensity of the potential fallout and embarrassment), they can persuade victims to give them money or explicit pictures and videos to prevent them from doing so. Setting aside the illegal nature of this kind of thing, especially if the victim is a minor, the bully can subsequently receive even more material from their victim which can be used to further harass, intimidate, and embarrass them.

Social media can cause problems to grow exponentially. If it's a slow news day, even a minor issue can spread and become common knowledge very quickly. This isn't a phenomenon limited to children, either; a lot of adults are the victim of cyberbullying. With such volatile circumstances representing the norm of the world our children are growing up in, it's essential that we understand how to effectively deal with all types of bullying so that we can help our children to manage the trying experiences they're likely to be confronted with at some point in their lives.

How to Deal with Bullying

When your child is being bullied, you're faced with a very difficult and specific situation. The circumstances of bullying vary significantly, meaning in turn that the best response in any given situation must be at your and their discretion. When you find out that your child is the victim of bullying, the first thing you should do is give them as much reassurance and love as you can. Remind them that their whole family loves them and will support them; they're not alone, and they will get through this. People are horrible, and kids can be especially cruel, but nothing lasts forever. There are always options for you to take to improve the situation.

Making the school faculty aware of the situation is one of the first courses of action for most people, and it can be effective in many cases.

However, when the school can't or won't act in the necessary way to mitigate problems, things get more complicated. Likewise, it can be extremely difficult to get the police involved in any way that will be productive, but if laws have been broken then this may be an option for you. If the school and the police aren't able to assist you and your child is being badly bullied, you can consider moving schools or otherwise getting them away from the source of the trouble. If it's milder and they think it will pass in time, your child might be prepared to put up with teasing for the present time. After all, moving schools is a traumatic experience in and of itself, and there's no guarantee that things will get better. Having to leave all of their friends behind and start over again is often something that many children just don't want to do.

Another factor to consider here is that in the age of the internet, moving schools isn't guaranteed to be all that effective. It's possible that your child might move only to find that the entire school district already knows about something that happened at their old school and the bullying simply starts again. This is a depressing state of affairs, I know, but it's the reality of the world we live in, and if you're going to help your child confront their problems you have to break everything down with them and assess what their options are in a pragmatic and realistic manner.

When confronted with the knowledge that their child is being bullied, many parents have an understandably angry and proactive response such as going to speak to the parents of the bullies or confronting the bullies themselves. I'd urge caution to anyone considering this course of action; it can be effective in some circumstances, but it can also just end up making things worse for your child, particularly if the parents of the bullies aren't reasonable or understanding people. I'd recommend similar caution for those who tell their children to fight back. Again, realistically this can be effective in some circumstances, but it can also make things far, far worse and can escalate the bullying to a higher level of intensity, making a relatively small problem much worse.

Grey Rocking

One of the best techniques there is for dealing with bullies or any form of conflict in which the victim can't immediately remove themselves from the situation is called 'grey rocking'. This is essentially the process of being as neutral, unprovocative, and emotionally withdrawn from the perpetrators as possible in order to minimize the response they get from bullying. When people are bullying others, they're doing it primarily for the reaction they know they will get. They feel powerful at being able to dominate and control others who they see as weaker than themselves, often to compensate for some aspect of their own life where they feel out of control. Grey rocking is a tactic most commonly used to bore stalkers, psychopaths and narcissists into moving on to another target for people who are on the receiving end of their maladaptive behavior. It can also be used to good effect against bullies, however, as their motivations for doing what they do are similar.

They're looking to control and hurt. They want a certain response from their victims, and grey rocking can deprive them of this. When their behavior suddenly brings them little or no satisfaction, bullies will often just move on to a different target. It's tough, but it's the way of life. Grey rocking means making yourself as boring and emotionally neutral as possible. For example, if your child is being called names and teased or rumors are being spread about them, applying the grey rock method would mean not reacting to any of it — not saying anything back, not letting them know they're hurt by what's being said, just acting as neutral and unbothered as possible, as though it were happening to someone else entirely, and then getting on with their lives and their studies, and enjoying the company of people they like. This can be difficult to do at first, particularly when the bullies are physically violent or threatening, but over time it becomes easier to do and more effective. Without the response and control and ability to hurt that keeps them thriving, bullies tend to get bored.

Of course, the course of action you decide to take in response to your child being bullied will vary depending on the exact circumstances of their situation, and the correct call is whatever you decide is best.

What to do if Your Child is Bullying Others

This is a situation that many parents don't consider and for good reason. No one wants to believe that their child could be capable of making another child's life a misery, and most of us I'm sure would think that their kids are too well raised to behave that way. The truth is that anyone can be a bully at some point in their lives. We each have the propensity for it written into our genes. It's important to understand how to handle such a situation just in case it ever arises.

First, you should do your best to understand why your child has been bullying other children. Communicate with them to work out why it's happening and what you can do to address the root problem. Without doing this, the problem will probably continue, as your child will continue to feel the need to exert their power over others. If you can get your child to open up about why they're doing what they're doing, you can work together to solve the underlying issues they're facing and stop them from taking out their frustrations on other people.

Finding a better outlet for their pent-up feelings can help, too. You then need to make sure your child fully understands the gravity of their actions and how much pain they can inflict through bullying. If you can do this and help your child to view their actions with a new outlook, they will likely feel remorseful and seek to make amends on their own. If they don't, it may well be your place to make sure they do this so that you can draw a line under the whole experience, learn from it, and move on. Leaving problems unsolved can lead to resentment festering and could even have future consequences for your child, so do your best to make sure all parties involved at least speak about it and your child apologizes, as well as ensuring the behavior stays curbed for good by remaining vigilant.

Discipline And Boundaries

Behavior correction is a fundamental part of parenting. Children tend to be unruly and mischievous. It just comes with the territory of being young, curious, and not knowing any better. Raising a child involves shaping them by teaching them to know better, and this requires instilling healthy amounts of discipline in them and setting strict boundaries. Doing this in a positive way isn't any more difficult than harsher, more traditional methods, and it leads to vastly improved results across the board. We need to implement family rules in order to give our children a clear framework of what kind of behavior is and isn't acceptable. Without these well-enforced boundaries, children are more prone to acting up and causing trouble. There is a certain sense of calmness that comes with a child understanding what the rules are and how they are expected to behave. For children that lack this clear framework, it can often feel they their behavior is punished arbitrarily. If their parents aren't consistent, how can they be expected to have a good idea of what they're going to be punished for and what they can get away with? The result tends to be kids that simply do what they want and worry about the consequences later. Do your best to explain to your children why the rules are there and why they're fair, even when they're wholeheartedly convinced that a 'certain rule' is an opposite of fair.

The first step in cultivating disciplined and well-behaved children is to clearly establish what they can and can't do, and why. Explaining the reasoning behind the rules will help tenfold with their enforcement — children tend to accept things more easily when they make sense. If you can show them how the rules are there to keep them safe and keep the family sane, you'll find they'll follow them with far less difficulty than if they're just the rules 'because I said so, that's why'. Setting out all the rules you need to enforce in an exhaustive list isn't possible, so teaching your kids why the rules exist and the reasoning behind them helps them to decide for themselves whether or not something they're doing or considering doing is acceptable behavior or not; this helps them to think and act in a more responsible manner.

Introducing these rules into your home will depend on the ages of your children and the level of development that they're at when you begin to properly introduce and enforce them. If you have young children, this might just be a matter of teaching them the ropes as they go, gently telling them what is and isn't acceptable as and when things occur. If you haven't explained that a particular rule exists yet or why because it simply hasn't been a problem before now, then it's a good idea to give children a warning to let them know that there's a rule there that needs to be followed rather than just immediately punishing them, or they will (quite rightfully) deem it unfair and be more likely to act out. If you have older children, however, then it might be a good idea to draw up a list and have it somewhere clearly visible in the home to serve as a reminder of what behavior is and isn't acceptable to help make the transition to a clearly defined boundary structure easier for them.

The nature of childhood will mean that your children have issues with rules. Infants of nearly any species of mammal are more playful and unpredictable than their adult counterparts as this playfulness, energy, curiosity, and spontaneity makes the steep learning curve that comes with being young easier to handle. Generally speaking, unacceptable behavior should be a small slice of your children's experience of life in order to allow them as much freedom and enjoyment as possible. Some people would prefer that their children not to run and jump around at home, but doing this can deprive our kids of the things that, at their age, are the most natural and healthy things in the world, just because they're inconvenient to us. Positive parenting is therefore about setting out healthy and fair boundaries for our kids to make sure they're not out of control while also avoiding the frustration of keeping them on a leash for most of their young lives. Compromise is important here; you might allow your children to run and jump around (providing they're careful) at certain times, but that doesn't mean it has to be permissible under all circumstances. For example, if you have guests over, or you're trying to unwind in the evening, you want your children to be calm and collected. You have to figure out how to balance rules and a sense of order with your children's happiness and enjoyment of their lives by taking their and your needs and wants into careful consideration and working out guidelines that work for everybody in your own family.

Part of setting effective boundaries in your home is avoiding falling into the trap of becoming a permissive parent. Don't try to avoid inciting anger and tantrums by steering away from confrontations and letting your children get their own way. Doing this will only result in your children having poor emotional development and regulation. They'll expect to always get their own way and go ballistic when this doesn't happen. Children from permissive families tend to be far more rebellious and antisocial than those with families with good boundaries and discipline.

Reinforcement: Punishment and Reward

When you're trying to get your children to stick within the boundaries you've set for them, enforcing the rules consistently is equally as important as making sure they're aware of what they can and can't do, and why. Enforcing the rules doesn't have to be about shouting or excessive punishments or threats or terrifying your children into submission. The concept of discipline in the context of positive parenting is based on a concept that is firmly rooted in behavioral psychology: reinforcement.

The idea behind reinforcement is relatively simple. Essentially, correcting behavior is simply a matter of conditioning your children to want to do good, positive things by rewarding them when they do those things while dissuading them from doing disruptive and negative things by punishing them when they misbehave. This is known as reinforcement — you're showing your child that certain behavior leads to certain and consistent outcomes, either positive or negative. You're reinforcing the link between their behavior and consequences in their mind. It's as simple as that; the real skill is in the application of this concept. For example, if a child is refusing to go to sleep when it's their bedtime, you have two different avenues of approach. You could either tell them that they need to go to bed or they will be punished, such as by grounding them for a weekend or taking TV or toy privileges away, or you could say that if they go to bed now they will be rewarded, such as by taking them out for ice cream on the weekend or going to the park.

There are therefore multiple options that can be taken to get the child to behave and get the job done. A key aspect of this system is that you need to follow through with what you've said you will do. Using empty threats without substance and failing to keep your promises for rewards will only serve to teach your child that what you say isn't to be trusted and that they should, therefore, do whatever they want, as they're unlikely to face consequences or be rewarded. You have to stick to your guns. If you threaten your child with punishment and they continue to misbehave, you must follow through with it, even if you don't want to.

Just because you're punishing your children doesn't mean that you can't do it in a positive manner, either. It is entirely possible to only punish your kids in a loving, understanding way while keeping the desired outcome of the punishment — behavioral correction. The trick to doing this is to avoid acting out of anger, malice, or frustration, but instead thinking things through in a measured and considerate fashion. Giving yourself the opportunity to reflect and calm down before you decide on their punishment out of anger and have to backtrack is a good idea. For example, if one of your children is misbehaving and it's driving you up to the wall, you can send them to their room to give you a chance to cool off and decide what their punishment should be. Then, when you're ready, go up and talk to them, gently explain why their behavior is unacceptable, and inform them of their punishment. Doing this consistently will ensure that your kids learn to take you seriously and respond immediately to your warnings because they know that you mean what you say and that you will follow through with punishment.

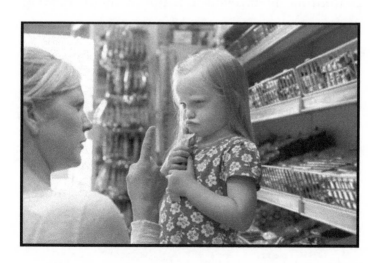

A lot of parents struggle to implement positive parenting techniques when their kids are being especially difficult, such as when they're flat out refusing to listen to or obey their parents or they're acting out, being aggressive, and possibly even violent. Parenting positively in situations like this can be very challenging, but it is possible. A point that needs to be made here is that no one is perfect, and everyone loses their temper sometimes. If you find yourself shouting at your children when they're being especially difficult, don't beat yourself up about it. Parenting is difficult enough without making yourself feel guilty for doing what comes naturally to you and won't harm your children in the long run, provided it's not a regular occurrence.

Sometimes it can be necessary to raise your voice and become stern in order to show your children that you mean business. In general, the underlying respect that comes with positive parenting should help to avoid this being much of a problem with your children once you've really gotten into the groove of things. If your children are being particularly difficult and hard to control, then the punishment you decide on should be more severe in order to really ram home the point that such disobedient behavior is totally unacceptable and will not be tolerated. Again, you can do this in a positive manner by clearly explaining to your child why you're doing what you're doing, why you had to raise your voice even though you don't like doing so, and how if they wish to avoid similarly strict punishments in the future, they should listen to you immediately when you tell them to do something.

Behavior management in positive parenting is therefore about commitment and understanding why your child is doing what they're doing as well as why you're doing what you're doing at every step of the corrective process. If you know why your child has been especially difficult at a given time, you can take steps to ensure this is mediated in the future. For example, if your child has had too many sugary drinks or too much candy and becomes wild and out of control as a result, you can avoid allowing this to happen again by letting them have sugar in moderation. Often, children act up because they want attention. This is especially true in large families or those with parents that are particularly busy. Once a child works out that they can get the attention from you that they crave by misbehaving, they're conditioned into doing it again and again — because it works every time. If you attend to your child before they have to resort to dirty tactics to get your attention, you'll have an easier time reigning them in.

Manipulation

Children can be crafty at doing this kind of thing; they tend to understand more than they let on. If they can work out ways to manipulate your authority, a lot of children will use them. For many kids, this comes down to using their charm and their wit to catch their unsuspecting parents off guard and get what they want from them without them even realizing they've been played.

A classic example of this would be a child playing their parents against one another in order to get what they want. They might lie and tell their dad that mom has given them the green light to eat more cookies, or they might wear down a particular parent with repeated tantrums and fits when they're alone but act like a perfect angel around the other one in order to upset the balance of power and have some amount of control stemming from the different experience each parent gets of their child. Often, children

143

attempting to manipulate their parents will go for the weakest link in an attempt to break the unity their parents share. They might hone in on their dad because they know he's easier to coerce into getting what they want. This is why it's vital that you stand your ground as a team and refuse to give in, no matter how effective the manipulation might seem to be. If you don't give them what they want, they will eventually realize it's a waste of time and energy.

Another example of manipulation is children that will use negative or aggressive behavior in order to control you. They might throw tantrums to get what they want, either at home or in public where they know you're more likely to cave and comply because they're making a scene and you're embarrassed. Some kids will decide they don't want to go to bed, and that there's nothing you can do to make them. They'll scream, cry, throw things, punch and break things, and hurt themselves in order to control you. In this way, you can find you're little more than a puppet whose strings they know exactly how to pull. Never give in and give your children what they want when they're trying to manipulate you using tactics like this. As soon as you do, they know they're onto a winning formula. Once they know that you will cave if they persist long enough and cause enough damage, it can be extremely difficult to coach this manipulation out of them.

Making sure you handle attempts at manipulating your authority properly is the key to staying a step ahead and avoiding being brought down to their level by participating in power struggles, which allows you to parent positively even in the face of challenging circumstances. The truth is that there are no power struggles unless you let there be. Your child is a child, and you are their parent and an adult. You are responsible for them, therefore you have authority over them by default. Your love and compassion for them are what creates the potential for them to exploit you to get what they want. If you were a worse parent, they wouldn't even have the opportunity to play their games in the first place. Your children can try to subvert your authority all they want — it will only work if you let it work. Never give in to tantrums; go straight home with them if you have to, and once they've calmed down make sure they understand their behavior is totally unacceptable. Punishments should be appropriate, here. If you have to ground them for a couple of weeks to get the message through that you will not tolerate manipulation and power struggles, so be it. If they throw more tantrums to protest the punishment, extend the punishment for as long as necessary until they realize they're fighting a losing battle. Then, stick to it. Don't give an inch, no matter how nicely they begin to behave in order to try and get back into your good books so that you end the punishment early. Positive parenting means you discipline and punishes with love — but you still need to do it. If you fall for the nice-guy act, you'll be right back where you started the next time they don't get their way and decide to throw a tantrum. The only way to break the vicious cycle of manipulation is to make a stand and show them that you will not back down and that tantrums will only lead to serious consequences for them and not what they want.

Reinforcement Step-By-Step: Punishment and Reward

Here's a useful step-by-step guide to cultivating good behavior through punishment and reinforcement.

1. Identify and label the behavior

When your child behaves in a way that gets your attention, ask yourself what it was and why you noticed it. Was it because they're behaving well and you're proud, or because they're misbehaving?

2. Warn or praise them

Decide how you should proceed based on your initial assessment of the situation. If the behavior was positive, then praise your child for behaving well and let them know you've noticed and appreciated their good behavior. You can even tell them that they'll be rewarded if they keep it up to really encourage them. If their behavior was negative, tell them so as firmly but softly as you can. Once your child is aware of how you operate and knows you stick to your word, it shouldn't be necessary to shout at them to get them to comply. Give them a warning not to do it again, and make it clear that if they do there will be consequences. Emphasize at this point that they have a choice as to how they will behave, and if they choose poorly they will regret it. If you're specific with the terms of the warning, make sure it's something you're prepared to follow through with to avoid making empty threats.

3. Punish or reward them

If your child continues to behave well, reward them somehow. This doesn't have to be anything special, but it should be something they enjoy. Going swimming, to the movies, getting ice cream, or even something as simple as a hug, telling them you're proud, and making them peanut butter and jelly sandwich while they watch some cartoons or play with their toys can be effective. It's a good idea to scale the reward with their behavior to save the best rewards for when you're really blown away by something they've done and want to show them how great their behavior was.

If your child has been misbehaving and continues to misbehave after a warning, punishment is the next step. Like rewards, the punishment you decide to use should scale with the severity of their misbehavior. It should never be malicious or stem from a place of anger or a desire to inflict distress. Depriving them of something they like to do can be an effective measure, as long as it's reasonable, fair, and won't impede their development. Grounding, sending them to their bedroom, time-outs, and taking away rewards can all be useful tactics here, but try to avoid performing the same punishment repeatedly every time to keep the novelty of it alive.

4. Allow them time to reflect and/or cool down

After you've informed your child of their punishment or reward and have begun to carry it out, give them some time to mull things over, calm down if necessary, and think about how they behaved and whether or not the result of their behavior was good or bad. This cooldown period is especially necessary when you're punishing your child because they're very likely to be upset and wound up. Give them space to breathe and be by themselves for a while.

5. Explain why they're being rewarded or punished

This is an important and often overlooked part of the reinforcement process. Without this explanation, you won't give your children the opportunity to really learn from their mistakes and successes, assess where they went right or wrong, and make a firm conviction to maintain or alter their behavior going forward. Once they've calmed down or otherwise moved on from the initial state of mind caused by their behavior and subsequent punishment or reward, approach them and gently lay out to them the reason you took the action you did, how you felt about their behavior, whether you're happy and proud or disappointed, and how you expect them to behave in the future. Make sure to praise them if you can, whether it's for calming down and being good after misbehaving or maintaining good behavior.

You should also take this opportunity to reassure your child that you love them, especially if they're being punished, and to tell them that you take no pleasure in punishing them but you have to do it for their own good.

6. Ask if they understand why they were punished or rewarded

After another pause to allow time for your previous explanation to sink in, ask your child if they understand why you did what you did to see if they've learned their lesson. If you sense that they still don't fully grasp it, try your best to gently explain it once more to ensure the point is reinforced.

Through the use of this method over time, you will notice real, tangible positive differences in your child's behavior, no matter how badly behaved they are.

Developmental Behavior And Age Specific Tools

In this section, we'll be looking at how your child's needs and behavior will change throughout the course of their lives as they progress through the different stages of their development. We'll outline exactly how to handle specific situations and difficult circumstances that will arise as a result of this, giving you an in-depth understanding of how to parent in a positive way no matter your child's age.

Infants (0-12 months)

Infancy can be an overwhelming stage of your child's life for you, particularly if you're a new parent. Despite the terror that comes with the humbling and profound realization that you're now completely responsible for a totally helpless, tiny human being, at this point in your child's life the main things they need from you are your love, care, and support. They're totally dependant on you, but as long as you're attentive and care for them as much as possible, you're doing all you can and should do.

An infant can seem very different from your conception of what a human being is at first. They're unable to do anything for themselves other than sleep and cry. However, your infant child is every bit as conscious as you — they just lack the mental and physical equipment they need to interact with the world in the same way as you. Virtually everything they sense and interact with for the first few months of their life is a complete and utter novelty to them. Your role at this point in your child's life is to act as a caregiver and a secure base from which your child can explore the world and learn about how to be human.

Every bit of love, affection, and attention you give to your child during this stage of their life will have a real influence on their development going forward, so make sure to cuddle, touch, talk to, laugh with, and play with them as much as you can. Don't worry about spoiling them, either. The faster you respond to their crying, the less they will cry for attention — making your life easier as a result. At this point in your child's life, the greatest difficulty they present tends to be waking you up in the middle of the night whenever they feel like it.

Toddlers (12-36 months)

Once your child is a toddler, things really begin to take off. This is a period of rapid development that sees them going from a relatively consistent and predictable baby to a little person teeming with personality. Once your child has learned to walk and talk, you start to really have your work cut out for you as a parent. This period of their life is a time of rapid development, cognitively, socially, emotionally, and physically.

Positively parenting children this young can be a challenging experience at times. Toddlers are famous for their plan-shelving meltdowns, where they decide that the only thing on the agenda today is a screaming tantrum over anything and everything. Children this young are only just coming face to face with their emotions for the first time, so they're understandably bad at regulating and processing them. Even minor inconveniences or perceived unfairness such as them getting a different type of candy to their siblings can quickly descend into a spiraling sort of chaos, even if the type they have is their favorite and they don't want what their siblings have. It's often about the principle, and once they've decided they're going to scream and cry all attempts at calming them down can quickly become ineffective as they will only dig their heels in further and keep themselves upset no matter what you do.

Positive parenting emphasizes cultivating understanding, empathy, and patience for your kids, and these things are especially important when raising a toddler. Understanding your child's motivations at this age is about learning how to guess at their internal thought processes and desires by carefully monitoring and reading their words and behavior. Toddlers represent a unique stage of childhood where they're just beginning to learn how to behave like they see everyone else behaving around them, while also wanting to indulge their own desires. You can generally see meltdowns coming in the stages beforehand, so if you're attentive you can avoid some of them with some quick thinking and problem-solving. Unfortunately, however, you won't be able to dodge all of them, and plenty of screaming, red-faced tantrums are to be expected from any toddler, usually when they don't get their own way.

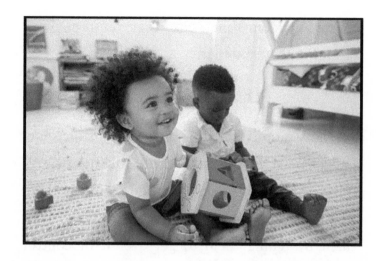

Toddlers are difficult because they're just discovering their own autonomy and independence. They're slowly working out that they have a level of influence over the world and people around them, and they're eager to exert that influence to get their own way. They want to exercise their will and have things the exact way they want them to be. When that doesn't happen and their preferences aren't met, they're prone to quickly resorting to a meltdown. Responding to these tantrums is difficult, especially when you're in public or you have a headache or you're trying

to handle something else that requires your
attention then and there.

The most important thing to keep in mind when
you have a tantrum-throwing toddler is that how
you respond to their emotional meltdowns will
influence how they cope with the same emotions
that cause them in the future. If you respond to
them by telling them to get over it or control
themselves, they will only become more
distressed. They can't control their emotions yet
- that's why they're having meltdowns in the first
place, so saying things like this will only make
the problem worse. We shouldn't minimize our
children's emotions or encourage them to bottle
them up, but rather encourage them to be
expressive of how they feel. This might seem
counterproductive, but research from Arizona
State University has shown that kids who are
allowed to express their emotions by their
parents tend to be more socially aware and less

angry. In the same way, children that are punished for their negative emotions are usually far worse at processing them; they don't understand or like the fact that they're experiencing them, which makes the problem worse.

Instead of punishing children for meltdowns, it's better to coach them calmly, thoughtfully, and compassionately on how to process and regulate their emotions in a healthy way. This will lead to less intense meltdowns in the future and a better emotional balance for your child. Once a toddler has started having a meltdown, it's very difficult to get them to stop. There's no easy fix for this other than just giving them what they want, which is never a good idea because they'll be more inclined to just throw a fit every time they want something. You, therefore, have to be patient, wait for them to calm down, and try your best to help them understand why they were so upset and walk them through how to handle their emotions better.

Here's a step-by-step guide on how to do this:

Step 1: Stay calm - this is more easily said than done when your child is screaming and crying, but it's absolutely vital for you to remain in control of yourself and be as collected as possible in order to get a grasp on the situation.

Step 2: Acknowledge how they feel - empathize with your child. Tell them that you know it's hard and that it's okay that they're upset. Let them feel heard. Let them feel understood. When you don't dismiss your child's feelings, they tend to calm down more quickly.

Step 3: Take them aside - if possible, remove your child from the situation in order to give them some breathing room. You can take them aside, take them to their bedroom, perhaps. Just let them get some breathing room away from whatever or whoever upset them, if possible.

Step 4: Wait for them to calm down - at this point, you've done all you can to speed things up. All you can do now is wait for them to calm down, however long this might take. Some children take longer to calm down from a heightened emotional state than others.

Step 5: Validate their feelings - you have to show your child that it's okay to feel how they're feeling. If they hear that it's okay to be upset, the frustration they might feel at being upset will evaporate fairly quickly.

Step 6: Coach them on their behavior - show them a better way to handle the problem they've encountered than just throwing a tantrum. For example, if they're upset that they didn't get enough juice in their cup, you can explain to them that they can simply ask for more. Show them that this will solve their problem far more effectively than just breaking down in tears.

Step 7: Show them, love - give them a hug and tell them that you love them. This will both help them to feel better by boosting their mood and show them that your actions came from a place of love. They will have a better understanding of how to react to their emotions and feel good for you have reacted the way you did.

Another great tip for managing toddlers is to be mindful of how you phrase things. Toddlers are highly sensitive to this kind of thing, especially when it comes to their independence. Giving them two options with the same outcome where one of the options allows them to do something for themselves can make your life far easier. For example, you can ask them if they'd like to get dressed or if they want you to help them. The freedom of choice and independence this kind of phrasing provides for a child makes a lot of potential tantrums easier to avoid. Once you've got a good handle on managing meltdowns, caring for toddlers becomes easier. Hang in there, keep your cool, and keep practicing the above method to gradually coach your children out of the tantrum phase and cultivate better emotional regulation.

Children (3-10 years)

The post-toddler years of your child's life will take them through a broad spectrum of growth and development over a long period. You won't notice much change day by day, but a child at four years old is a gulf apart from the same child at ten. During this time, your child's emotional and cognitive development will mature from a little boy or girl just out of diapers to a young person with their own well-developed interests, opinions, and way of seeing the world.

Parenting through this stage of your child's life involves helping them grown into the young person they're becoming. You'll see them start preschool and elementary, and witness all the developments, large and small, that come along with them. You'll still have meltdowns to manage from time to time, especially early on, but your role here gradually shifts away from being a caretaker as your child becomes more and more able to look after themselves. You might no longer have to bathe or dress them, but you will get to be there to listen to how their day was at school, help them with their homework, and give them advice about the life they've only just started living. You can help them understand others and coach them on making friends and getting on well with others.

The emphasis here is on facilitating and guiding their growth to prepare them for adulthood. As their cognitive and emotional development enhances their ability to comprehend the world around them, your child will be increasingly able to appreciate and learn from your wisdom. You can teach them how to share and enjoy the company of others, how to deal with loss, setbacks, failure, and grief, especially as they encounter situations that are the hardest thing they've ever had to endure by a long way such as the death of loved ones, trouble with other kids at school, and not doing as well as they'd like to have done in sport or class. Positive parenting here also involves preparing them to handle success in a beneficial way, as well as failure. The values you demonstrate to your children here will be instilled in them and reflected throughout their lives.

Understanding your child's motivations at this stage of their life becomes more complicated as they become better at hiding their thoughts and feelings. For the most part, children at this age are interested in having fun and enjoying their lives, which make these years, in particular, a beautiful time in their lives that you can take an active part in and enjoy along with them. As your child slowly matures, it's a good idea to give them the opportunity to make more and more of their own decisions in order to prepare them for adulthood. If they want to do something that you might not agree with, give them the opportunity to make their case. If they can convince you that what they want to do is in their own best interests and are capable of explaining why, it's a good idea to let them do it — as long as any risks are mitigated, of course. This will help them to mature and take more responsibility for themselves and provides them with the critical thinking skills they'll need in later life.

Preadolescents (10-13 years)

After the relative stability of childhood, parenting preadolescents begins to once again represent a very challenging chapter of your life as a parent. This period of your child's development brings a whole host of challenges and anxieties to their life, which will directly influence how they treat and react to you as their parent. Chief among your concerns when approaching how you handle parenting at this stage should be the growing level of independence your child needs and wants. Many parents find it difficult to accept that the baby they've raised and nurtured for so long is growing up into a young person, and are understandably cautious with the level of freedom they grant to their child. However, seeing as the transition from relatively little independence to total independence is going to have to happen eventually, it's a good idea to get off to a good start by addressing these concerns and ensuring your child is responsible enough to make their own decisions while also keeping a watchful eye on them as they begin to mix with new people and become exposed to different influences.

Your child's friends will begin to have a greater and greater influence over your child at this age as their priorities make the natural and inevitable shift from what their parents think to what their friends think, especially when they begin middle school. You'll likely notice them becoming closer with friends and wanting to spend more time out of the house at this age, so do your best to make sure they're making good decisions and choices and hanging out with people who are a good influence on them while also giving them the room they need to breathe.

In order to understand your child's motivations at this age, think back to your own experiences of this time. It was likely filled with a lot of uncertainty and expectation, and pressure to keep up appearances and conform to the norms of your peers in order to fit in. You might have felt self-conscious about the way you looked and dressed, or the things you did in your free time, or worried about your family embarrassing you if they were seen in public with you. Understand new challenges and anxieties of your child's life as you can, and try your best to give them space they will increasingly need while leaving the door open at all times for them to seek your advice, love, and reassurance.

Adolescents/teenagers (13-18 years)

Following on from preadolescence, this stage is most often classed as beginning with the onset of puberty in your child. This on its own brings a whole host of complications, issues, and anxieties into their life that you must try your best to help them with. This is without a doubt the most trying period of most people's young lives, so more than ever here your child needs your guidance, understanding, and sensitivity. Your child at this point will begin to resemble the young adult they will soon become, but they lack any of the self-assurance or confidence that they will hopefully possess in the near future. They lack experience with virtually every aspect of adult life that they've suddenly been thrust into, and for the most part, are just making it up as they go, so they'll look to you to assist them as they navigate a new and confusing world.

High school, especially, can be hell on earth. The petty drama, gossip, and superficial values make it difficult to navigate without a lot of stress, all of which will happen while your child is trying to pick their way through minefields like exams, acne, puberty, and burgeoning relationships. They're likely to be stressed and frustrated a lot throughout their teenage years, with the hormones coursing through their veins causing mood swings and shifts of perception that make certain events much harder to deal with. You'll catch your fair share of flack and bad moods throughout these years, which you have to try your best not to take personally while gently reminding your child that you are there to help and support them and you're only trying to do what is in their best interests. Never allow yourself to be spoken to or treated with disrespect, but have compassion for the difficult nature of life at this age at all times.

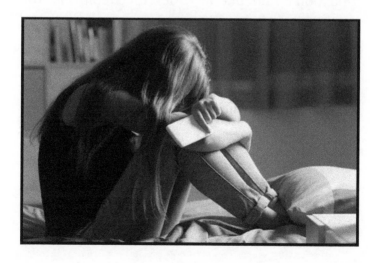

A teenager's motivations can vary wildly. By this point in their development, the emotional and situational complexity of their day to day lives can begin to resemble your own. Sex and relationships will begin to become a part of their existence, which is something you need to make sure they're educated and prepared for. Whatever your own attitude towards the place of these things in your child's life, you have to respect their growing autonomy and the fact that if you try to control them they will very likely rebel and do things anyway and just make sure you don't find out in order to circumvent the problem. With this in mind, you should embrace the idea of your child discovering their own sexuality and try your best to support and guide them to make positive and healthy decisions with this new aspect of their life. Whether you do this or not, they're going to be making their own decisions regardless, so it's a good idea to make sure you still have input and can provide advice by not shaming them or trying to control what they do.

Exercise: Positive Parenting In Action

1. Objectively assess your children

Get a pen and some paper and write down the names of all of your children. Then, underneath each of their names, try to list some things that come to mind about them. Think about the problems they might be facing, stressors they might feel in their everyday lives, that kind of thing.

Once you've written these notes, read them back and reflect on them. Try to work out how you could be a more positive parent for them, how you could be closer to them, perhaps, how to have more positive interaction with them and be a deeper part of their lives. Think about the relationship you have with them and how it could be improved from both sides; what each of you would need to do in order to forge a deeper bond between the two of you.

2. Listen

Take the time to have conversations with each of your children where you try to listen far more than you speak. You can start off by talking with them about anything but try over the course of the dialogue to press deeper into their lives and find out what problems they're facing that they might not have mentioned to you yet.

Doing this will help you to form a better understanding of the lives of your children and the problems they're facing. You can then see how what they say to you compares with the notes you've written. You'll probably find that you're surprised by how much you didn't know. When we really take the time to listen to our children, we learn who they really are.

Part Three:

Defining Your Family Culture

Every family is made up of the individual bonds between its members. Collectively, these relationships generate an atmosphere that engulfs the whole family unit — a mood or tone that sets the background of any interaction. When you go out for a family dinner, when you wake up on a Saturday morning, or when you get invited to a wedding, your family atmosphere determines the dynamic your family has, the way in which you interact, and the way you feel about each other and everyone else.

The Family Atmosphere

The type of atmosphere your family has is a direct result of the relationships that you create with your children and any co-parent. If your attitude towards the members of your family is open, relaxed, loving, and understanding, then the bonds between your children and the atmosphere your family emanates will be, too. It will be the type of family that radiates joy, laughter, and kindness. Your home will be one of those where everyone feels loved and appreciated. It will be the backdrop for years of beautiful memories and happy times.

An open and loving family atmosphere provides a safe, constructive, and creative backdrop for your children from which they can learn, grow and explore the world. They will be able to live life at their own pace, in a way that is right for them. They will be encouraged and supported throughout all of the difficult moments of their young lives; their best moments will be shared with the people that matter the most to them in the whole world. While some parents will be lucky enough to have parents of their own who are as loving as they are and can contribute to a supportive family atmosphere, the extent to which you can create a good atmosphere depends entirely on the people that make up your family. For example, you might find that having a great atmosphere amongst the members of your immediate family is relatively simple, while things change when relatives and extended family are present. We can't pick our family, and some people are luckier than others when it comes to the relationships they have with the people in their families. If you have difficult in-laws or parents, or a sibling whose presence spoils the kind and loving atmosphere of your family, don't dwell on it. Focus instead on cultivating the best atmosphere you can for your children; who knows, perhaps one day you'll have grandkids, nieces, and nephews of your own and able to participate in a loving and peaceful extended family.

Your family atmosphere molds and shapes your children into individuals. It shows them what is important in their family. It tells them who they are, where they come from, and who cares the most about them in life. Your children learn from you, from each other, and from the atmosphere of the family. They learn how to behave and how to talk, what is permissible and what is not for them to do, and what attitude to have towards life. In this way, we indirectly influence the decisions our children make through the way we model our roles as people to them. An anxious and stressed parent will very likely raise an anxious and stressed child. The behavior and mannerisms of the people in your family transfer and imprint upon your children.

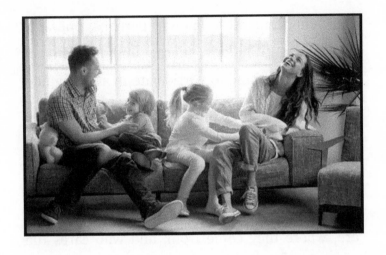

Some family atmospheres encourage cooperation and teamwork, whereas others set the stage for competition and conflict. As a parent, you are responsible for the atmosphere of your family. Through your attitude and actions, a whole field of meaning and purpose is generated and sustained by the members of your family. The mood of your family is a reflection of your principles and values. If you prioritize having fun and enjoying life above all else, your family atmosphere will mirror this. Your children will absorb these priorities and reflect them back at you, and your home will have a laid-back, relaxed vibe. Whatever standards you set, your children will follow. A pattern is therefore created by yourself and if you have one, your partner. The interaction you have with your partner will be observed and imitated by your children. If you're affectionate, emotionally open, and giving towards your partner, then your children will reflect these values, too.

Maintaining a Good Atmosphere

Making sure the atmosphere your family possesses stays positive, understanding, and supportive of all its members is a daily task. The atmosphere is only as good as the relationships between the individuals that generate it, so as a parent it's your role to make sure that any stress and conflict is handled in the right way. You can't stop bad things from happening to the people you love, but you can choose to approach any negative experiences with a mindset that seeks to learn any lessons there are to be learned from them and process your own emotions healthily.

This is the philosophy that is at the heart of any good family atmosphere. Your outlook is far more important than the actual circumstances of your life. If you're able to be positive even in the darkest moments, your family will feel positive and continue to be a place of mutual love and support no matter the difficulties you might be facing, because they will look to you in order to gauge how they should react. This is the reason that children whose parents consistently react to situations with fear and panic will be similarly nervous and panicky themselves, and will likely grow up to be this way, too. Your children model themselves on you by learning and taking their cues about how to behave in a given situation from how you react.

A great example of this is parents that panic and overreact when their child falls over. The child might be completely fine, but the fact that their parents are showing so much concern and makings a big deal out of things can teach them that they should be upset, and make them promptly burst into tears.

Maintaining a positive family atmosphere, then, is about cultivating a positive attitude within yourself. When you treat yourself and the other members of your family in a positive, respectful, and patient manner, they will reflect this attitude back both towards themselves and towards the other members of your family.

Familial Democracy

A family, like any organization, needs good leadership. It needs people to step up and demonstrate the right way to act and live life in order to set the tone and be the example that the other members of the family can emulate and learn from. Traditionally, families would have had one person who led it — often the man of the house, a patriarchal figure, who might even have continued to be the leader and shot-caller once his children had children. Matriarchal setups have also been common throughout history, particularly in families with groups of sisters.

As a parent, you get to decide how your family operates. An increasingly common concept these days is to run your family like a democracy instead of a monarchy. Rather than having one person or a few people who have the power and make the decisions, you instead treat everyone equally. Everybody has a voice, and everybody's opinion matters, no matter the subject. As a parent, you are still responsible, but you encourage your children to have their own opinions and state their case in a mature and rational manner.

Having a family dynamic of this kind has a number of benefits for your children:

- Encourages independence
- Promotes critical thinking
- Fosters self-reliance
- Allows everybody to be heard and feel respected and appreciated
- Closer bonds and better openness amongst family members

Running your family in a democratic manner will cultivate better bonds between the members of your family and allow your children to flourish no matter their personality or preferences. Family discussions are characterized by calmness and fairness, with everybody getting their chance to speak and everyone feeling able to be open and honest about what they think or how they feel. Having a family democracy is about more than letting everyone be heard; it's about treating everyone equally, no matter their age or personality.

Your children's confidence will be greatly reinforced by having the opportunity to speak their minds and be an individual, knowing full well that they will be heard and respected no matter what the conversation is. Healthy socialization like this allows them to become better adjusted to speaking to other people and will bring out their personalities in shining color.

Honesty, Trust, Mistakes, And Forgiveness

Being human is an inherently difficult and confusing journey. The circumstances of our lives arrange themselves into impossibly complex situations that make always doing the right thing very difficult. We aren't perfect. Everybody makes mistakes. it's simply human nature to mess up, to hurt the people you care about and be selfish. With this in mind, there are two attitudes we can take towards how we view the truth of the reality we face every day. Either we can dwell on our own and others' mistakes and allow resentment to sap away our happiness and joy, or we can accept that they're as much a part of being human as eating and breathing and that we wouldn't be who we are without them. When we take this latter approach, we free ourselves to be empathetic towards ourselves and others and to better understand the negative aspects of being human, rather than attempting to bury them or push them away.

We tend to judge others by their actions and ourselves by our intentions. When we shine the light of understanding into the darkest parts of ourselves, we learn that the truth of being human is that we are all of those things we fear. Within each of us, no matter how good or how pure we might seem to others, is the potential to be the very worst versions of ourselves possible. This dark side is as much a part of ourselves as the light, as the kindness and the compassion and empathy. It's only once we realize this that we can begin to approach the mistakes the people dear to us make with a different point of view. Deep down, everyone wants to be loved, accepted and understood, and when we make mistakes and hurt the people close to us we isolate ourselves and push them away.

Part of building a positive family culture is learning to accept that each of us will make mistakes and each of us will, in turn, need our love and forgiveness. Family is the one thing in this world we can count on when the chips are down. The only truly unconditional love is the love that close family members have for each other, where no matter what, no matter how badly our children or our parents or our siblings mess up and make mistakes, we are able to come together, accept any apologies, and offer our love and forgiveness. When everybody in the family understands that they will always be a part of the family no matter what, they are free to truly be themselves.

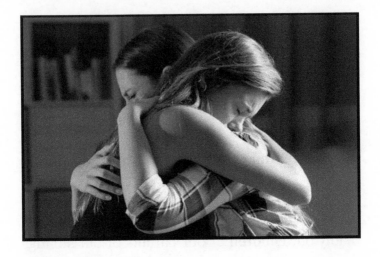

If you're going to parent positively, if you want to cultivate a family atmosphere of unconditional love and acceptance, then you have to live in a way that places a tremendous amount of importance on honesty and trust. You have to sculpt your family into an open and accepting group to belong to, where everybody feels like they can be themselves and that they can trust their fellow family members with their life. If you want your family to be honest and to trust each other, you have to put the work into creating the accepting atmosphere that would allow openness and honesty to prevail. That means having an understanding attitude and patient manner that allows people to speak up and own their mistakes without fear of being shouted at, rejected, or resented. For example, if one of your children gets into trouble at school or breaks something precious to you, they will only feel able to own up to their wrongs if they know that they can safely do so without fear of retribution or malicious punishment and shouting.

There needs to be a mutual understanding between every member of your family that honesty with each other will always be valued, no matter the consequences. Prioritizing being open with the truth over punishing people, especially when they know they've done wrong, will lead to a beautiful family culture of forgiveness for each other's wrongs, big and small. At the end of the day, when someone knows they've messed up and truly, deeply regrets their actions and feels remorse for what they've done, they are punishing themselves far worse than they could ever be punished by anyone else. When people feel hurt by someone else, they often bear a grudge and want punishment for the sake of it, to make the other person feel bad. This is seen as justice, as an eye for an eye. Some parents will react to their children making mistakes with anger and physical violence, not realizing or not caring that the point of punishment isn't to hurt and avenge but to teach. We punish children in order for them to learn about what is right and what is wrong. If they know they have done wrong, then an open and honest conversation about it will do far more to rectify the mistake and heal any wounds than making them feel even worse through punishment.

When you build relationships with your children that are based on these positive values, with the understanding that they will always be loved and that there is no wrong they can do that it would not be better to simply be honest about rather than hide, you push yourself towards new heights of acceptance and understanding, and forge bonds with your kids that are based on sturdy foundations of deep and profound love and respect. These are bonds that can be built on and expanded over the course of lifetimes, the relationships we most cherish and will go on in our children's memory and legacy for their own children and their children's children.

When mistakes are made and arguments occur between the members of our family, a culture of forgiveness is essential to mending bridges and healing rifts. Fights between family members can be brutal — there are few people in the world we know better and therefore few people in the world we can pierce more scathingly with just a handful of words. We can hurt each other terribly because we know each other inside out and we know that we're family so we can treat each other poorly without ruining relationships forever. People can become deeply hurt and scarred from these conflicts, so a culture of forgiveness is absolutely necessary in order to heal deep wounds.

Building a firm foundation of absolute trust, especially between parent and child, is an integral element of creating a warm and loving family culture. A child should be able to tell their parent anything and have total confidence that their parent will both keep that information safe and act only in their best interests. Cementing this bond of trust is one of the keys to positive parenting. It is at the core of the parent-child relationship, something that remains constant and consistent throughout childhood and beyond. Developing this trust isn't something that can happen overnight. Like any trust, it stems from year after year of reliability and consistency. It's built when you clean and apply a band-aid on their scraped knee, and when you get them out of a tricky situation with their math homework. It comes from you acting in good faith and with love towards them for an extended period of time.

The Family Journey

L ife is a journey, but not one where the destination is the goal. If this were the case, the only point in life would be dying, and there wouldn't be time to enjoy the music, art, beauty, and laughter along the way. The journey itself, rather than the destination, is the point of life. It's a journey we ultimately have to make alone, but that we can share with certain people for certain stretches of it. The true beauty in life is that we can build our family around us in whichever mold we wish, in order to have like-minded loved ones to share all of the joy and laughter of life with. Your family will take its own journey through life as the individuals that make it up to walk their own paths and share the experiences they have with one another. Your children's journeys will in this way be influenced by your own.

Understanding Your Journey And Accepting Yourself

As a parent, you are the central component of your child's development. Your personality, attitude towards yourself and others, and your outlook on life will all directly influence the person your child becomes themselves. Like the key to your child's emotional growth, cultivating a loving and understanding relationship with yourself is vital in order to build and maintain the same thing with your child. If you respect, accept, and love yourself, your children will mirror you and have those same qualities for themselves in abundance, because the lessons you've learned from a lifetime of experience will be available for them straight off of the bat.

Living your life in the best way possible is first and foremost about having a good relationship with yourself. Through this, all things are possible. Without the ability to understand and forgive yourself, you'll go through life unable to take responsibility for your decisions and therefore restrict yourself to living out a shadow of the life that you could have experienced. If this is your fate, it will be the fate of your children, too. They will learn from you how they should feel about themselves. When they see you upset and angry that your life hasn't worked out exactly how you might have wanted it to, the lesson that they will learn is that they cannot expect to ever be in control of their own happiness. They will come to expect to always be the victim of the circumstances of their lives, rather than being empowered to accept what they must about themselves and their lives and creating meaning, purpose, and enjoyment on their own terms. That's why it's essential to learn to love and respect yourself — for the sake of your children, as well as your own happiness and inner peace.

Having a good relationship with yourself means completely forgiving yourself for your mistakes, past, present, and future alike. It means being able to feel angry, and stressed, and guilty, and ashamed, without feeling ashamed of feeling that way in the first place. When you understand that your life is a riddle of ever-increasing complexity, when you see that you cannot ever expect yourself to be anything other than the flawed human being that you are, you gain the ability to let the weight you carry around with you everyday slip off of your shoulders. Just like happiness, accepting yourself is an attitude, not a state of affairs. It's not about periodically stopping to confess your sins and forgiving yourself for them, but forgiving yourself for your mistakes at the moment, right as you're making them, even when you're aware you're doing something wrong and will continue to do so in future. This attitude towards yourself will rub off on your children through the way you behave and the things you say, and they too will come to understand that they can never hope to be perfect themselves or have perfect lives, and instead that all they can do is try their best to enjoy all that is good in their lives without dwelling too much on what is bad or what mistakes they have made.

In addition to the lessons, your children will learn about how they should treat themselves just from knowing and interacting with you, having a greater understanding of yourself will enable you to be a better parent for them, too. You will be more empathetic, more aware of, and better at accounting for their own internal trials and tribulations when you're faced with challenging situations as a result of the private battles raging in their own lives, no matter how trivial they might have once seemed to you. Everybody is fighting their own battle deep inside of their minds.

When you have respect for yourself, you will have greater respect for others, including your children. Your children will have respect for you, too, as well as learning how to have respect for themselves. Respect is the cornerstone of any genuine relationship and is a vital ingredient in cultivating a healthy, loving bond between them and you. It paves the way for great communication and the transference of ideas and understanding between you and them. Without this two-way respect, they wouldn't sit and really listen when you speak, and you wouldn't feel the need or even that you had the ability to really help them learn the important lessons in life in the first place.

The Theory of Attachment

Children learn through observation and imitation. Whatever you do, they will pick up on, and internalize the same kind of thoughts and feelings that you express as part of their own interior model. As human beings, we tend to operate as what is essentially a collection of incredibly complicated patterns. We form habits and ways of thinking, feeling, and living based upon these patterns that set the tempo that we follow for the rest of our lives and can change only with a lot of effort and insight into ourselves. The mental patterns we form as children, therefore, follow us throughout the rest of our lives. There is no better example of this than the theory of attachment, a concept pioneered by the psychologist John Bowlby as a way of trying to understand how the experiences we have as children deeply influence our personal development and follow us throughout the rest of our lives.

The theory of attachment suggests that children need to form a physical and emotional attachment to a caregiver in order to feel safe, secure, and at ease. This allows them to have a safe base from which they can explore the world and interact with the people around them without fear or anxiety. Bowlby's theory states that children who don't form a secure attachment with a caregiver when they're young have far more troubled and emotionally bleak lives than those that do. They grow up to represent a higher percentage of crime and violent crime figures than children who are securely attached. This goes to show the importance of the experiences we have as children in influencing what the rest of our lives will be like.

The habits your children form and the patterns they internalize will follow them throughout their lives. For this reason, it's important to give them as securely attached an emotional base as you can in order to let them grow and flourish.

Having as good a relationship with yourself as possible will enable you to do this for them.

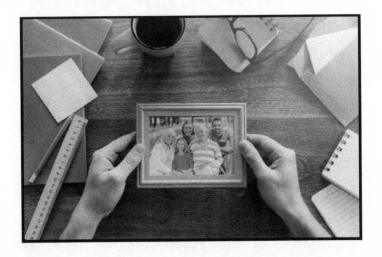

The Importance Of Attitude And Perspective

Your whole family's journey is shaped by their (and by extension your own) attitude to and perspective on life. There is no more important factor in determining the quality of the life you live than the mindset you approach your every waking moment with. Your outlook on life will affect everything you think, do, and say, and has far-reaching consequences for your family's legacy and future. For this reason, a fundamental part of positive parenting is to try and develop a positive outlook on your life and the lives of your family.

This is far more easily said than done, of course. We've all watched self-help videos on YouTube or read books about how to have a more positive outlook on life and worry less. The harsh truth is that often, we have a minor uptick in mood, motivation, and positivity afterward that gradually gives away to the same crushing disappointment with the circumstances of our lives as soon as we're slapped in the face with reality once more. It's difficult to stay positive when everything feels like it's crumbling to dust all around you. It's hard to remember not to stress when there's a difficulty at work and we're worried about our jobs and how we're going to put food on the table and provide for our children.

Managing Stress and Coping With Adversity

So, how do you stay positive in a world that looks so negative so much of the time?

Here are some of the main difficulties that people face in life, and what attitude you should try to approach them with in order to have a better outlook on things, as well as some practical solutions towards mitigating the negative effect they have on you.

1. Stress - stress is the natural response we feel as a result of being exposed to things that pose a threat to our safety and security and the wellbeing of our family. When we're scared, our body goes into something called 'fight or flight' mode, where the essential survival functions of our bodies like our ability to run, think, and fight are prioritized at the expense of less immediately important ones like digestion or sleep. This is all well and good when you're trying to fight off a predator, but when you get a bill in the mail at the beginning of the month that you can't pay and you're behind on rent and your child needs new shoes, it's not quite as effective. Stress is corrosive, especially when it's present for long periods of time, as it tends to be in our highly stressful modern lives. It takes a toll on us mentally and physically, wearing us down inside and out, raising our blood pressure and making our hearts work harder to keep us alive and healthy. Stress can be addictive. We can find ourselves learning to accept and normalize its presence to the extent that something feels wrong when we don't feel stressed. Obviously, this isn't a state of affairs that's particularly conducive to enjoying our lives or having a positive or healthy outlook on things.

Dealing with it - when you're trying to shape how you view the stress you feel in your mind, it can help to remember that it's there for a reason, but it's been hijacked by a body that doesn't know the difference between the imminent threat of death and bills being unpaid. The level of stress you feel more often than not doesn't correlate with the real difficulty you face, no matter how much it might feel like it does. Knowing this won't help to pay your bills or put food on the table, but it will help you to put the way you feel into perspective and help you to relax somewhat. No matter how stressed you are at the situations in your life, you're going to be alright. You will survive, you will keep your children fed, and you will keep on going. You will find a way out of any situation. Think back to times in your life when you felt extremely stressed over something that now seems minor and insignificant. Chances are, you don't even think about it anymore, and your brain has moved on to being stressed about something else. In the future, whatever you're stressing about now will probably feel as minor and as insignificant as those things in the past do now.

It's important to give yourself the time and the space to unwind. You need to take care of yourself in addition to your kids. Make sure you allow yourself the breathing room you need to have peace and quiet be a regular part of life. Some of the most valuable advice I've ever been given was to remember to create myself a life that I didn't feel the need to constantly escape from. You can do this yourself by prioritizing your own mental health and taking time to de-stress whenever you need to in whatever way works best. Some people find this in having a bath and a glass of wine, others in going for a walk or hanging out with their friends. Do whatever you need to do to avoid yourself constantly feeling drained, and don't feel guilty for needing to do it.

2. Worry - This is the gnawing feeling you get in your gut that something is about to go very wrong, and you desperately need to avoid it by coming up with a solution. Just like stress, however, the level of worry we feel often doesn't correlate with the true scope of the threat presented to us in the situational problems of our lives. Worry serves its purpose only when it prompts you to think about what you can do to mitigate a problem. At all other times, it's just an unnecessary burden that prevents you from enjoying your life. Like stress, worry can be addictive. We can come to feel it so often and so intensely that it feels wrong to be without it. I know that many people, like myself, have experienced that awful, surreal feeling of being worried that they don't have anything to worry about and end up desperately searching for the next thing to latch onto and agonize over.

Dealing with it - Try to shift the role you see worry as having in your life. Rather than seeing it as necessary in order to protect yourself and your loved ones, attempt to view it as the largely unnecessary and enjoyment-sucking parasite that it is. Sure, sometimes you have good reason to be worried, but for the most part, you don't. There is only what you can do and what you can't do in response to a situation. If you can do something, do it. If you can't do anything, then there's nothing to do but let it happen. Whatever way you look at things, worry doesn't make it any better. It just takes all the color and peace out of life, and if you're not enjoying your life, what's the point in being so worried about it? You have nothing to lose. Try to just accept that what will be will be, do what you can, and don't fret over the things you can't control.

Some practical solutions for reducing anxiety include trying to anchor yourself in what's going on in the here and now by allowing yourself to become completely absorbed by the company of your friends and family, a book, or a movie, or music. Take the time to focus on the positive aspects of your life. When you feel the anxiety rise up inside you and beg you for attention, close your eyes. Don't push it away. Don't respond to it, either. Just let it be there, acknowledge that it's there, and then go back to what you were doing before with your full attention. It's okay to feel anxious, but if you can stop yourself from responding to and indulging it whenever you feel it rising up, you can break the vicious cycle and stop yourself from giving in to the urge to worry whenever you feel it.

3. Money - This is one of the biggest stressors in the lives of the vast majority of people around the world. Everybody wants more money, everyone feels like they don't have enough, and everyone is trying to work out how to get more of it. You need it just to survive; you can hardly even take a step without needing to pay for something, somewhere. Money is important, but it's not all there is to life. If you have enough to survive and get by without living in poverty, you're better off than most. This offers little comfort when you haven't got enough to take your kids to the movies or buy them nice presents for the holidays, but it's good to keep the relativity of it in mind. Even if you had more money, you wouldn't necessarily be happier. Lots of people come into money and find their happiness even decreases. When you expect money to make your life better on its own, you give your power to enjoy your life over completely to an abstract concept.

Dealing with it - It's difficult, but if you can shift the attitude you have towards money, you can find satisfaction in the things you have rather than dwelling on those things you don't have that could be brought into your life if only you had the money. There's no one size fits all quick fix to situations where you're in desperate need of money that anyone can offer you, but you can find ways to make money if you think creatively. Remember that all of the things that really matter in life are within your grasp already. As long as you're with the people that matter to you and having fun, you have everything that truly has meaning already. That's something that money can't buy.

4. Time - Many people feel like they don't have enough time to really enjoy their lives. It's such a common theme that we look for desperate ways to make the most of things, often depriving ourselves of precious sleep in order to meet all of our commitments. The problem is, there will always be something to do. There will always be places to go and people to talk to that put demands on your time. You have to realize that there will never be enough time in your days or your life to do all of the things you need to do.

Dealing with it - Instead of rushing around doing the things that you need to do, you should prioritize the things you want to do instead. Life is short. What point is there in spending it all trying to meet the demands that are placed on you if you leave no time to actually sit back and enjoy yourself? Be honest with yourself about how longs things will take. Make time for the things that matter to you the most, and drop those things that you don't care about. Life is too short to spend any more than you absolutely have to on things that don't fulfill you.

You can only pay attention to so many parts of your life at once. Whatever you pay attention to, you tend to get sucked into. You see all of the associated thought branches and rabbit holes that lead you on until you're lost in the middle of it and don't know how to escape. Learning to manage the stress and adversity you face in your life involves learning to balance the different parts of your life and make sure you're paying attention to the right ratio of good to bad. Dwell on the bad only as much as you have to; make sure you take care of what you can and learn any lessons there are to be learned and then let it go. If you can focus on the good, you will have a much fuller spectrum of the rich tapestry of life to enjoy. Family days out or evenings to become a treasure, rather than another chore to complete. You only get to live your life once, and it will be over sooner than you realize. Fully enjoy and appreciate all of the positive things in your life rather than taking them for granted by honing in on the negative. Focus on sharing your part of the family journey and living it to the fullest extent.

Sharing Happiness

Happiness can seem like an elusive concept sometimes. It's slippery. It tends to hide from you. Happiness is, a way of looking at the things in your life. That's all. It's about appreciating what's there to be appreciated — and there is always a lot there to be appreciated. This way of looking at things will enable you to find the hidden joy and beauty within your life. Try to keep up a positive state of mind, because the way you perceive the world creates the reality you inhabit on a daily basis.

One of the best ways to appreciate the beauty in your life is to share it with other people, and there are few better people to share happiness with than your children, as a family. Have you ever watched a comedy movie or stand-up show on your own and noticed that you barely even laugh? If you do, it's probably just blowing air out of your nose with a bit more force than usual. If you were to watch the same thing with the people close to you, you'd find it way funnier. Laughing is a social activity. We just don't find things as funny when there's no one to share the joke with. Being with the people we love the most is what life is all about. Love is where the true meaning of things lies. Spend the time you have with your family and friends while you can, because they won't be around forever.

Exercise: Defining Your Family Culture - Self-Assessment

1. What is your family culture like?

Ask yourself what kind of atmosphere your family generates. Be honest, and write down some notes if you need to. Is your family happy, laidback, and supportive, or is the atmosphere in your home more negative and stifled.

Once you've reflected on what characterizes your family culture, think about how you'd like it to be different and what things you can do to get it there. Maybe you'd like it to be more open and honest, in which case you'd be proactive in demonstrating those values by opening up to your family about your thoughts and feelings.

2. What characterizes your personal attitude to life?

Take the time now to reflect on your own outlook and attitude towards your life. Do you feel satisfied? If not, why? What things would you want to change about your life? What aspects of your life are you unhappy about?

Ask yourself what you can do to change your mindset and improve your attitude to life. How can you enjoy it more? Perhaps you find you're always distracted, so you decide to spend more time with your family and pay closer attention to what's happening when you're with them, rather than being off somewhere mentally, thinking about something else instead of enjoying your life as it unfolds in front of you.

Final Words

With the lessons that this guide has provided for you, you're now ready to set out on your journey towards parenting in a more positive way. The way in which you raise your children is always unique to every family and every parent, but with the concepts outlined in this book, you'll be able to combine your own methods and practices with positive and healthy practices that lead to a happier, calmer way of life for your whole family.

Parenting positively means understanding that your children should be treated with love, compassion, and kindness at every turn. It means understanding that understanding itself is the key to forging deeper, stronger connections with your children; understanding yourself, understanding them, understanding your partner or co-parent, and understanding life.

You don't have to have a full understanding of any of these things in order to parent positively, only grasp that this understanding is the truly important thing. Having total understanding is not possible, so instead, we should simply strive to learn and come to understand more than we do already.

We have to learn how to interact with and talk to our children many times as they grow and change before their very eyes. It's not uncommon to look at them one day and realize that while they're still the same person, they're very different from the child they were just a few years ago. Being a positive parent involves re-assessing your tactics and the way you treat your children to meet the needs of their lives at whatever stage they're at.

Raising your children with these positive values means adopting the right attitude towards every aspect of your life, from the way you see each day and each person you know and love to the way you see yourself. Without an open, reflective, honest attitude, you cannot hope to prioritize the right things in life. You need to value all of the things that make parenting a beautiful and positive experience in order to internalize them and therefore radiate them into the people around you. It isn't enough to just want to raise your children positively. You have to want to live in a positive way, too.

This positive philosophy, when you really take it to heart, is apparent in everything you do. It's there when you listen to your child talk about the coloring they did with their new crayons and tell them how much you like the way they've used the different colors together. It's there when you reassure them and tell them it's okay as they're crying into your shoulder. It's there when you have to send them to their room and go to check on them and have a talk ten minutes later. It's there when they see you talking and laughing with them at dinner and they realize that everything that matters to you most in life is right there in that room.

Taking on the journey of parenthood isn't something that can be taken lightly. It's a huge responsibility; you're tasked with overseeing and managing the life and development of a small human being. But you don't need to worry about whether or not you'll do a good job, whether you're equipped with the right skills or whether you'll mess it up. Good parenting, positive parenting, is an attitude. It's an outlook on things, nothing more. When you have the right outlook, you're constantly looking to be the best you can be. It's why you bought this book, and it's why you're a great parent.

When you find yourself overwhelmed and frustrated, and confused about how to act in a positive way when it feels like your children just won't respond, remember that life is a journey of continuous learning. You're going to make mistakes, and you're going to learn from them. Sometimes you have to make a mistake before the solution to the problem you were struggling to tackle in the right way presents itself.

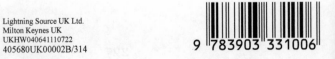